TRAVELING LIGHT

TRAVELING LIGHT

*Contentment
Amid the
Burden
of Life's
Expectations*

KURT D. BRUNER

MOODY PRESS
CHICAGO

To my parents,
who did more right than they know.
Thanks for the
years of hard work
and selfless giving.
I was blessed to be part
of your quiver.

CONTENTS

Introduction   9

Part One: Life's Expectations
1. Great Expectations?   15
2. Making Ourselves Poor   33
3. The Myth of Happily Ever After   55
4. When Everything Isn't Enough   73

Part Two: The Practice of Contentment
5. The Lost Art   87
6. The Impact of Identity   99
7. The Power of Perspective   111
8. The Curse of Comparison   127
9. The Gift of Gratitude   141
10. Making Ourselves Rich   151

INTRODUCTION

Never before have so many, who have it so good, been so unhappy. We are the most pampered generation in history, but we seem the least content. Our needs are met, our desires fulfilled, still we are not satisfied. Life has never been better. Living has never seemed worse. What is wrong with us? Why, in the midst of our indulgence, do we experience so little happiness?

I remember spending time with my grandparents as a boy. They were simple people who expected little from life. Having survived the Great Depression, they knew the meaning of sacrifice. In my childhood, "doing without" meant watching black-and-white television. In theirs, it meant going to bed hungry. Yet, despite their struggles, they always seemed grateful for and content with the basic provisions of life. They demonstrated a deep sense of satisfaction that was common to their generation and foreign to mine. They had fewer comforts and more strife, but they were happier. Why?

As I watch my two young boys play today, I can't help but wonder whether they will be happy in adulthood. I work hard to provide them with a nice home, warm clothes, and the other basics of life. I spend time playing, talking, and laughing with them each day. But are these things enough? My father's generation assumed that being good providers and faithful family men was the extent of their duty, only to face accusations of inadequacy from their adult children. How do I know whether my own children will look back on my efforts with gratitude or disdain? What can I do today to help them find happiness tomorrow? How can I help them become more like my grandparents' generation than my own?

I am convinced that the key to happiness in life has little to do with our standard of living, economic stability, or physical well-being. It is not dependent upon what our parents did, what our friends do, or what fate may bring. We are not unhappy because life is bad. We are unhappy because we expect too much. No life, regardless of how good it is, can measure up to what we want. Our generation has been a victim of something far worse than economic collapse or physical disaster. We have been convinced that life is bad because it is not ideal. We have sacrificed contentment and joy on the altar of fantasy. We are victims of our own expectations.

Let's face it. We bring nothing with us into this world, and we'll take nothing out of it when we leave. So we might as well learn to travel light in between. How? By managing our expectations and mastering the art of contentment. It makes little sense to burden ourselves with expectations that may or may not be fulfilled. We set ourselves up for the inevitable fall of disappointment.

Stated simply, disappointment is unmet positive expectation. Something good was supposed to happen, but didn't. As a result, we feel a sense of loss. In many cases, the loss can be severe—even devastating. Though no tangible loss is experienced, the impact can be all too real.

Jane married her high-school sweetheart at a young age. She now spends her days cleaning, feeding, and changing diapers—romance is only a distant memory. Her dream of "happily ever after" turned out to be nothing but a fairy tale.

Ron took a chance at his dream. He sold everything and gave up his job to launch his own business. Things didn't go as planned because the local economy went through a downturn. Now he's broke, feels like a failure, and has lost confidence in his own abilities.

John and Linda are a young couple in their late twenties. Like many of their friends, they are still driving an old car and scrimping to save enough money for a down payment on that first home. They are starting to wonder if they will ever reach the standard of living they were raised to expect.

Lisa has difficulty identifying with her pastor's series on building a healthy family. She has a family, but she can no longer even imagine it healthy. She worries about her alcoholic husband, Mark, and his influence on their two sons. She wants the boys to become responsible young men, but their model of manhood is less than ideal. Despite her efforts to keep the boys in church and teach them right from wrong, she fears that they will follow in their father's irresponsible footsteps.

The stories are endless. The feelings are the same. For some reason, life does not turn out as expected. As a result, we carry the heavy baggage of disappointment along with us throughout life's journey. Disappointment can quickly turn to disillusionment, disillusionment to hopelessness, and hopelessness to bitterness. Anger and heartache fill the void left by unmet expectations.

Yet unmet expectations are the norm in life, not the exception. More often than not, dreams remain dreams, goals are unfulfilled, and hopes mellow with the passage of time. It is only in the movies that a happy ending is standard fare.

Don't get me wrong, I fully believe that dreams can come true and that we should seek the best in life. I have experienced things in my own life which have far exceeded my wildest expectations. But like you, I have also experienced the disappointment of failed plans and abandoned hopes.

Happiness should not be measured by the dreams we've attained. It really is possible to choose joy and contentment despite unmet expectations. The days of excitement are relatively few, but disappointment is part of our ongoing experience. Real life rarely measures up to fantasy—or even to our dreams of having the good things it seems "everybody else" enjoys. Dealing with that truth is key to finding contentment in life.

How do we protect ourselves from disappointment while holding onto our dreams?

When does healthy anticipation become unhealthy presumption?

How do we balance working toward our goals with accepting our lot in life?

When does contentment cross the line and become complacency?

These are just a few of the questions we must explore in order to find a balance. We must maintain a drive toward excellence in living, while learning to accept reality. We must cope with disappointment without losing hope. Some have mastered this balancing act; many have not. I invite you to join me on the trip of discovery.

Oh, by the way, don't pack much. We plan to travel light!

Part One

LIFE'S EXPECTATIONS

Chapter One

GREAT EXPECTATIONS?

Our necessities never equal our wants. Benjamin Franklin

The best way to make a man poor is to increase his wants. The best way to make him miserable is to confuse his definition of happiness. Both are cruel, and both describe what we have done to ourselves.

The human experience has been revolutionized during the past century. We moved from an agrarian society, dominated by farm life; to an industrial era, dominated by factory life; to an information age, dominated by media and technology. We moved from needing to wanting to having—from surviving to producing to possessing. Our standard of living has never been better.

Unfortunately, the same cannot be said about our way of life. We are an unhappy people. It appears that the seeds of our destiny were also the source of our dissatisfaction. Something happened while we were pursuing the good life that robbed us of our ability to enjoy it—and we never saw it coming.

THE DAY OUR WORLD CHANGED

Once upon a time the citizens of our nation were generally content with and grateful for the basic provisions of life. Most people lived on farms, requiring long hours of hard work just to survive. But that was OK, because they expected no more.

But gradually an industrial revolution took place. It wasn't called that at first, nor did people fully understand what was happening. Slowly but surely, however, new things were invented and produced which could dramatically alter people's way of life. But most people paid little attention to all that. They were too busy with life as it was and saw no need to change it. After all, what could be better than owning land and working it with one's own hands? Life was good.

And then, one day, something happened. A man named Sears came up with an idea. He sent a catalog describing hundreds of wonderful products to every possible home on the prairie. Without warning, the average American farmer was confronted with the things he didn't have: better tools for his work, new gadgets for his home, fancy clothes for his wife, and exciting toys for his children. Once the spectacular world of merchandise entered the home, the simple life was no longer enough. How could anyone be satisfied with basic provisions when so many other things were possible?

On that symbolic day Americans' corporate expectations shifted from the desire for basic provisions to an endless stream of material possessions. They took the first step away from content living toward the never-ending pursuit of the good life. What they had was no longer enough. They had made themselves poor.

ANOTHER DAY

Many years later, just about the time most people had acquired the things they wanted, something else happened. Another "catalog" hit American homes. It seemed harmless enough. The television, at first a novelty item, became the vehicle through which a whole new world of possibilities entered homes. It brought entertainment on demand, educated us about the world around us, and reminded viewers that life was not yet ideal.

In his excellent book *Amusing Ourselves to Death*, Neil Postman explores the impact that television has had upon our culture. He shows how we have robbed ourselves of the ability to think because we have reduced everything to ten-second soundbites and amusing images. We want to be entertained, not challenged. I be-

16

lieve that television has had an equally devastating impact upon the emotional state of our society. Its images have robbed us of the ability to be happy because we expect more than real life can offer. We want gratification, not contentment.

Gradually, television convinced us that life should be more, much more than it was. Basic provisions and material possessions were no longer enough. We needed to experience romance and excitement like those lovely people on the screen. They had wealth, youth, adventure, health, beauty, and luck. Happy endings were the norm, and the good guys always won. A new standard of happiness had been set. We began expecting real life to compete with fantasy.

Sadly, this dynamic has affected every aspect of our lives. We are not happy with our relationships, our jobs, our standard of living, or our religious experience. We redefine happiness, placing it out of reach in the process. We make ourselves miserable.

WHAT HAPPENED?

Obviously, it would be overly simplistic to suggest that all of our societal dissatisfaction originated with the Sears catalog and the television set. They do, however, serve as important symbols of a larger movement which has been sweeping our world.

I am not suggesting that there is anything wrong with the level of wealth and comfort we've attained. In fact, I am a strong supporter of innovation and free-market activity, both of which increase opportunity and improve our standard of living. Nor am I suggesting that we become apathetic about our status in life. I believe that God is honored when man achieves his highest potential and that anything less is an insult to His creative design.

We should never be completely satisfied with our lot in life. Most of the great movements of history started with someone who was dissatisfied with the way things were. We have seen nations rise, diseases cured, technology advance, and repression overthrown—all because someone refused to accept life as it was. The pursuit of something better is good.

My concern is not over what we have achieved in life, but rather what we have come to expect from life. So much is possible in our society. And because so much *can* be, we somehow feel that it *should* be. As a result, we have lost appreciation for what is.

17

This is not a new problem. People in every age have found themselves disappointed by unmet expectations. For some reason, however, it seems far more prevalent in our generation. Although we are more blessed, we are less content. Never before have we had it so good. Never before have we been less grateful. Why?

THE POWER OF EXPECTATIONS

In his classic work *Great Expectations,* Charles Dickens created a telling example of how expectations can impact our lives, for better and for worse. The story was set in nineteenth-century England. It interwove the lives of several interesting characters—each of whom related in one way or another to young Pip, the key personality of the book.

The story began with Pip as a young orphan boy. He lived in the modest home of his older sister and her husband, Joe, the blacksmith. Although his sister was overly demanding and demeaning toward Pip, Joe was a hard-working and caring person who became Pip's mentor and best friend. As he grew, Pip served as Joe's apprentice and faced the likely future of becoming a blacksmith alongside a man he admired and loved. Things were turning out good for Pip despite the early setbacks of his life.

Pip was given the opportunity to periodically visit the home of a wealthy, heartbroken neighbor named Miss Havisham. She was a very strange, bitter woman who had put her life on hold years earlier after the man she loved failed to show up to their wedding—instead sending a note which ended the relationship. She lived alone with her beautiful adopted daughter, Astella, with whom Pip fell in love. The visits, originally designed as a service to Miss Havisham, became opportunities for Pip to see Astella. Unfortunately, Pip was repeatedly reminded of his inferior status, being merely a common tradesman rather than a gentleman with the advantages of education and wealth. Suddenly, what had been an honorable profession was no longer good enough for Pip. He began striving to improve his education in hopes of someday gaining enough wealth to become worthy of Astella's affections.

After years of hard work and diligent study with very little to show for it, Pip was discouraged. During a conversation with a close friend who was reminding him of how good his life had been, Pip insisted that his circumstances were inadequate. "I hate my life! I hate being a blacksmith! I've seen a different world. If I'd not been to Miss Havisham's, I'd be content with what I have."

It wasn't long before Pip's good fortune came. An anonymous benefactor endowed him with great wealth. He was sent to London to receive the best available education and social training. He purchased fancy clothes, plush furniture, and the finest foods. The honor and status he wanted became a reality. Pip was a gentleman. He was finally worthy of Astella's affections, and he could rekindle the happiness he had set aside in pursuit of his dream.

Unfortunately, Pip lost his beloved friend, Joe, after becoming too good to associate with such common folks. And the woman he worked so hard to impress married a man of greater wealth. He lost his joy when, in pursuit of great expectations, he lost the ability to enjoy the simple things of life. All that he ever wanted was not enough to fill the artificial void created in his life by those early visits to the home of Miss Havisham. His "great expectations" turned out to be not so great after all. He lost what truly mattered in the process < of getting what he thought he wanted.

Pip allowed high expectations to motivate him toward improving his education and status in life. That is good. However, he also allowed them to warp his priorities and steal his joy. That is bad. Expectations can affect us in both ways. Learning to benefit from the good without embracing the bad is an important step in dealing with our own great expectations.

EXPECTATIONS—GOOD OR BAD?

Some of the greatest accomplishments in human history have been motivated by high expectations. Henry Ford's famous Model-T helped shape the course of the twentieth century, all thanks to someone who diligently labored to perfect the internal combustion engine. The deadly disease polio has been virtually eliminated because one man spent years working to discover the cure. It was considered impossible for any human to run a mile in under four minutes, until one day someone did the impossible in the fervor of competition. Our once vast globe has become a small world due to significant advances in the telecommunications industry, which all started with a man named Bell who refused to give up on an unlikely idea. History is filled with examples of people who were not content with the status quo and who broke free of traditional boundaries as a result. Holding themselves to a higher standard, they raised the human experience to a new level.

Unfortunately, high expectations can also be the source of some very bad things in life. A husband leaves his wife after a few years because he expected more from her than she could possibly give. A woman becomes bitter with God because He has not given the physical healing she expected in response to her persistent prayers. A pastor resigns his church after ten years of ministry, severely discouraged because the congregation didn't grow as he expected. Disillusionment often becomes the bitter aftertaste of high expectations.

We are left to wonder whether expectations are something good that we should nurture or something bad that we should repress. Should we embrace them or avoid them? Should we pursue them or ignore them? The answer is both. The key, as in many areas of life, is achieving balance.

In one way or another, the things we expect have a significant impact upon every part of life—our response to situations, our relationship to others, the goals we pursue, our spiritual walk, the things that motivate us, even our worldview. It is impossible to separate what we expect from what we do. Although we may not always fully understand how our expectations influence our attitudes and actions at any given moment, their effect is nonetheless real.

Expectations can bring either positive or negative results in our lives, depending upon what we do with them. They can result in positive discontentment which motivates us toward improvement, or negative discontentment which pushes us toward disillusionment. By identifying some of the consequences of our expectations, good and bad, we may find it easier to achieve the balance required to help foster the former and avoid the latter.

POSITIVE EXPECTATION

All discontentment is not necessarily bad. Total contentment with all circumstances may not be entirely good. The things we expect should motivate us toward improving our circumstances or altering our attitudes. These are what we will call "positive expectation." By understanding the good influence of discontentment, we

20

can better manage the "great expectations" which come our way. Let's examine several potential benefits of discontentment.

Vision

Expectations can help us see past the way things are to the way they could be. They prevent us from being satisfied with the status quo by giving us a vision for something better. Nothing great has ever been accomplished that did not begin in someone's mind as a vision of what could be.

In his best-selling book _The Seven Habits of Highly Effective People,_ Stephen Covey says that those who accomplish much do so because they begin with the end in mind. In other words, before beginning the journey they map out where they want to be or what they seek to achieve. The ability to see beyond the present reality and envision a future objective enables individuals to improve the world. Those who are unable to see past difficult circumstances and obstacles toward a better tomorrow will remain trapped by the limitations of today. Winifred Newman said, "Vision is the world's most desperate need. There are no hopeless situations, only people who think hopelessly."

In this context, expectations can have a positive impact in our lives. They can serve as the catalyst for a much-needed vision of what life could be, which is a critical first step toward a better day.

Ambition

As important as it is to have a vision for tomorrow, seeing the possible is not enough. Millions of people have a vision of what life could be, only to become discouraged over their current status. Rather than being a target for the future, their vision becomes a point of comparison for the present. In order to avoid this common trap, we must allow our expectations to foster a healthy dose of ambition. We should establish aggressive goals and create a plan of action for reaching them. Ambition helps us turn our vision into reality rather than pie-in-the-sky fantasy.

Some people have no vision or ambition to move forward in life. In fact, they generally see high expectations as the enemy of contented living. As a result, expectations do not prod them toward setting and achieving goals. They passively accept whatever life may bring, good or bad, with no inclination to influence or alter their circumstances. They may think that they've attained an advanced state of contentment. Yet too often their attitude is really confusing contentment with complacency. True contentment gives us the ability to find fulfillment in the midst of circumstances that we cannot change. Complacency causes us to passively accept circumstances that we could change if we tried. The former is healthy, the latter is not. Unfortunately, many excuse complacency in the name of contentment—considering themselves more noble than others because they have no ambition.

Jesus told a story which demonstrates that passivity is a character flaw, not a virtue. In Matthew 25:14–30 He described a common business scenario. A wealthy man entrusted his assets to three junior executives, giving them each an opportunity to practice what they had learned in investment school. Each chose a different approach to handling the money. The first and second servants did well, doubling the value of what they'd been given thanks to some savvy investment strategies. The third servant, however, took a rather unconventional approach with his money. He was afraid of risk, so he hid it in an underground safety deposit box where it earned no profit whatsoever. Needless to say, his strategy did not impress the boss. "You wicked, lazy servant!" he yelled. "You should have put my money on deposit with the bankers, so that when I returned I would have received it back with interest." He then fired the passive employee, giving his share of the business to the more aggressive first servant. Jesus used this parable to teach a very important spiritual principle: We should make the most of the opportunities we've been given for God's glory.

This story is just one of many scriptural examples showing us that passivity is not a sign of spiritual depth. It is a consequence of laziness.

Motivation

Once we've seen what is possible and established goals to move us toward that vision, something must motivate us to keep going despite the inevitable setbacks and obstacles we will encounter. Our dreams and goals can be that source of motivation. Like young

Pip who determined to become a gentleman after seeing Miss Havisham's wealth, we can allow our own great expectations to push us through the difficult days and hard work required to make our dreams a reality. *encouragement* *Family*

Anyone who has ever run a marathon race knows the importance of motivation. Despite the months of diligent training to prepare for the big day, it is impossible to avoid intense pain and exhaustion during a twenty-six-mile run. The body reaches a certain point and starts to scream in agony, insisting that the runner has had enough and demanding that he quit. For some it occurs at five miles, others at ten, others at fifteen. Regardless of the precise distance, the same dynamic affects all marathon runners during the long, difficult race. This is why marathon organizers typically station people along every foot of the event with the sole purpose of cheering for the passing runners. They understand the important role of motivation to the process of endurance. As one marathon runner explained, though the people on the sideline may be complete strangers, there is something about hearing energetic cheers from others that motivates a person to push harder than might otherwise have been possible.

The same principle is true for all life endeavors. We can see possibilities and establish goals, but if we quit when facing pain or difficulty, then we accomplish nothing. In that moment when our spirit tells us that we've had enough and demands that we give up, we need something that will push us harder than we might otherwise go. We need something to cheer us on from the sidelines, motivating us to keep going. Our expectations can be that source of motivation. They can scream possibilities in our ear when we face discouragement, reminding us of the goal. They can refresh our spirit with hope when circumstances seem hopeless. Expectations motivate us by reminding us of the prize at the finish line.

Self-Improvement

We should never be completely satisfied with our own growth. The more we expect from ourselves, the more we will become. So it is best to allow expectations to push us out of our comfort zone, replacing the indulgence of self-gratification with the demands of self-improvement. Only then can we master the art of living.

We read self-help books, participate in Bible study programs, watch educational television, and talk to counselors, all to become better people. That is good. Our expectations help us zero in and address areas of ignorance, weakness, or sin—motivating us to increase our knowledge, ability, or integrity. For example, you may have picked up this book because there is an area of your life you hope to improve. You wanted to learn something that you didn't already know or focus attention on an area of your life with which you are dissatisfied. Either way, you are letting your expectations drive increased personal growth. Never stop.

Keep in mind that we must maintain balance when it comes to how much we expect of ourselves. William Ward was right: "Expecting too little of ourselves is wasteful; expecting too much of ourselves is folly." There is a point at which we can push ourselves too far. More often than not, however, we tend toward the other extreme.

If we let them, expectations can generate tremendous good in our lives. They can give us vision, foster ambition, motivate us through the tough times, and push us toward consistent self-improvement. In the effort to avoid the negative impact of our expectations, we must not lose sight of the positive things they can bring.

[handwritten margin note: Positive Expectations]

NEGATIVE EXPECTATION

Just as expectations can bring some positive things to life, they can also be the source of some very negative feelings and behaviors. If we let them, expectations can turn from motivating us toward improvement to pushing us toward disillusionment. Unfortunately, it is all too easy to let the negative overshadow the positive. But it doesn't have to be that way. By understanding the potential negative effects of expectations we can better guard ourselves from letting them rule our lives.

Dissatisfaction

While I was discussing expectations and contentment with a friend who works as a financial planner, he told an interesting observation. As part of his initial presentation, he routinely asks clients the question, "How do you feel about the level of wealth you've accumulated in your life so far?" He poses this same question to those who've amassed great wealth and to those who've saved virtually nothing. Almost without exception, he said, <u>those with little seem far more satisfied with their status than those who have much.</u> Surprising? Maybe not. Financial experts Joe Dominguez and Vicki Robin have seen similar results when they survey those who attend their financial-planning conferences. When asked to rate their overall quality of life, those with an annual income of more than $48,000 were less satisfied than those who earned $10,000 less per year. Even those with an annual salary of under $15,000 rated their quality of life higher than those in the top income category.[1] So much for the idea that more is better.

There can be a direct correlation between high expectation and low satisfaction. The more we get, the more we want. Those who have more are often those who have pushed themselves to get more. Unfortunately, they seem unable to enjoy what they have because it is never enough. This is the first negative impact of expectations. They can rob us of the satisfaction we work so hard to achieve.

I have found this dynamic to be true in more areas of life than just finances. After four years of diligent study and sacrifice, I graduated from college. Rather than rest in the satisfaction of that accomplishment, however, I went on to pursue a master's degree. After working up the ladder to a middle-manager position at work, I immediately set my sights on upper management. After realizing a life dream by publishing my first book, I set out to write a second. And so on, and so on. No matter what the accomplishment, the satisfaction never comes. There is always another hill to climb, another goal to reach. Unfortunately, our <u>expectations can deprive us of</u> an often deserved <u>sense of satisfaction</u>.

Stress

Robert Eliot gave us the secret to reducing stress in our lives. Rule number one, don't sweat the small stuff. Rule number two, it's <u>all small stuff.</u> Unfortunately, that is easier said than done.

All of us experience countless minor irritations in life that cause our stress levels to rise. These <u>irritations come</u>, in large part, <u>because circumstances fail to measure up to our expectations</u>. The idiot in the car ahead of you doesn't drive as well as he should. The weather is too cold, too hot, too wet, or too dry. (And if it happens to be "just right," you probably won't even notice.) The boss is too bossy. The kids are too loud. The pastor's sermons are too long. The grocery bill is too high. And the neighbor's dog uses your backyard as his personal restroom. And then, of course, you may also be facing some bigger issues—grief, loss, or disillusionment. Is it any wonder that you feel stressed?

I'm going to let you in on a little secret. The circumstances of life will never fulfill your expectations. Every day, in one way or another, something will bring disappointment or frustration. The key to reduced stress is not altering your circumstances, but rather altering your expectations. Why not learn to expect less-than-ideal situations since they are going to come anyway? Cut your family some slack by lowering your demands, and reduce your stress level in the process. Anticipate at least one idiot driver every time you hit the road so that you're not disappointed when you get behind him. Expect the boss to scream once in a while. You don't have to enjoy the minor irritations of life, but you can keep them from giving you an ulcer. You don't have to enjoy the major stresses either, but you can find ways to cope with them successfully.

When life fails to measure up to what we expect, we become anxious and our stress level rises. This is one more negative effect of expectations.

Selfishness

After only a few years of marriage, Bob and Kelly are on the verge of divorce. Like most young couples, they started out madly in love with each other. Oh, how things have changed. He is angry with her because the house is never clean enough, the Visa bill is never low enough, and their sex is never good enough. She detests him for spending too much time at the office, being too tight with the money, and giving her too little romantic attention. Bob and Kelly entered their marriage certain that they were made for each other. Now they are ending it because they see themselves as incompatible. In truth, they are experiencing one of the negative influences of expectations —selfishness.

When we become disappointed and experience hurt feelings in a relationship, it is often because we have placed expectations on the other person that he or she is unable or unwilling to meet. When

26

we insist that others meet our wants or needs without giving at least equal weight to meeting their needs and wants, we are being self-centered. Rather than adapting to the needs of others, we expect others to accommodate us. Instead of seeking to become a better mate or friend, we expect the other person to change. That, plain and simple, is selfishness.

Unrealistic expectations undermine healthy relationships. When we depend upon the people around us to meet our needs, fulfill our dreams, improve our standard of living, boost our self-esteem, and satisfy our yearnings, we are being self-centered. *If only they would change,* we think, *life would be better.* Think again. Jacob Braude wisely said, "Consider how difficult it is to change yourself, and you will realize what little chance you have of changing others." Our expectations do not improve other people. They only drive a wedge between them and ourselves.

Bitterness

Perhaps the most damaging consequence of unmet expectations is that they can drive us toward bitterness. If our dreams never come true, it is easy to become angry at God for giving us the short end of life's stick. After all, so the thinking goes, God could improve my circumstances if He really wanted to. Since He refuses to do so, I have the right to blame Him for my misery. Unfortunately, in our effort to punish God, we end up hurting ourselves.

The same principle applies in our relationships to other people. If others disappoint us and fail to meet the expectations we've placed upon them, it is easy to allow bitterness to fill the void created by our lost affection. Perhaps an old boyfriend or girlfriend broke off the relationship in the midst of your "happily ever after" expectations. Maybe your parents made some serious mistakes while you were growing up, and you can't bring yourself to let them off the hook by forgiving. Or it could be a grown child who rebelled against your values, a mate who abandoned you during his or your mid-life crisis, a pastor who violated your trust, or a boss who treated you unfairly. Whatever the specific situation, the impact is the same. We allow the failure of others to develop a root of bitterness in our heart, and we maintain the right to hate that person for what was done to us. But the destructive impact is in our own life, not the other person's. As

William Walton put it, "To carry a grudge is like being stung to death by one bee." We become miserable because someone else violated our expectations.

If anybody had the right to become bitter, Virginia did. Virginia was in her mid-forties, raising two teenagers alone because her husband had deserted the family four years previously. She could not drive because she had epilepsy, and the bus system in her city was unreliable at best. So to pay the rent and grocery bills, Virginia worked what jobs she could get within walking distance—one full-time and two part-time jobs. She worked late into the night at a fast-food restaurant, a job where most of her coworkers were high-school students. Her pay was little above minimum wage, and her boss regularly yelled at her because she wasn't as fast as the teenagers she worked with.

Yet Virginia was not known for her discouragement or her bitterness; rather, her gentle spirit was contagious. She took rebukes humbly, spoke of Christ when she got a chance, and produced high-quality work cheerfully. Her coworkers respected her, and some knew her as a model of unconditional love. In an environment where onlookers expect to see bitterness, peace is a pleasant surprise.

We must stop depending upon ideal circumstances for our fulfillment. We must stop depending upon other people for our joy. If we rely upon either to bring meaning to our lives, we will set ourselves up for a serious bout with bitterness.

FINDING BALANCE

We can ask ourselves several probing questions to help us begin moving in the right direction on the journey toward balance.

① *What do I expect?* As we will discus in chapter 2, we all have a unique standard of living against which we measure the circumstances of life. Creating a list of your personal expectations, the things you most want from life, is an important first step in learning to deal with them.

② *What can I influence?* Evaluate which items are within your realm of influence and which ones aren't. Next to the items which are largely beyond your control, mark "No." If there is something you can do to help bring it to pass, mark "Yes."

③ *What can I do?* If there are items you can influence, establish a plan for moving toward them rather than sitting back and waiting for them to come to you. Let your expectations motivate you toward bigger and better. Let them push you toward self-improvement where necessary. Overcome complacency with aggressive effort. Only then will you gain the benefits of positive expectation.

④ *What can't I do?* If an item is beyond your control, let it go. If you can't do it, don't depend upon it for fulfillment. That is not to say you can't hope, wish, dream, or pray for things to occur which are beyond your realm of direct influence. However, it does mean that you must trust, relax, wait patiently, and surrender your rights in the process. Doing so may not be easy, but it is essential if you hope to avoid the negative impact of expectations.

⑤ *What must I learn?* Finally, allow the things you have felt and experienced in life to push you into the classroom of contemplation. If expectations have undermined your joy rather than motivating your steps, do something about it. Be honest with yourself, and determine in your heart that you will grow where needed, change where required, and depend upon the Lord to move beyond the pain of disappointment into the wonderful world of contentment.

Young Pip's great expectations had both a positive and a negative influence on his life. Let's learn from his experience by finding the balance needed to keep the good and avoid the bad.

Know Thyself

No two people hold identical dreams and aspirations. Nor do we experience the same disappointments. So it is important that each of us spends time looking at our individual situation as we pursue contentment in life. We must evaluate what we've been expecting, locate our present situation on the map, and identify the primary obstacles we face in the quest for personal fulfillment.

In order to better understand your own level of satisfaction and contentment, complete the following personal evaluation. Be completely honest with yourself as you rate your present reality compared to what you expected from life. Circle the number that most accurately reflects your feelings, then add up your total points.

PERSONAL EVALUATION QUESTIONNAIRE

1. How satisfied are you with your present family life?

1	2	3	4	5	6	7	8	9	10
Not at all				Somewhat					Extremely

2. How often do you feel as though something is missing from your life?

1	2	3	4	5	6	7	8	9	10
Daily				Sometimes					Never

3. How do you feel about the content of your job?

1	2	3	4	5	6	7	8	9	10
Terrible				Tolerable					Terrific

4. How does your present income compare to your financial needs?

1	2	3	4	5	6	7	8	9	10
Way too low				Adequate				More than enough	

5. Compared to most of your friends, how would you rate your present standard of living?

1	2	3	4	5	6	7	8	9	10
Much lower				About equal					Much higher

6. How often do you struggle with feelings of inadequacy around coworkers, friends, family, and others?

1	2	3	4	5	6	7	8	9	10
Always				Sometimes					Never

7. How many of your longings, dreams, and goals have been fulfilled?

1	2	3	4	5	6	7	8	9	10
None of them				Some of them				All of them	

8. How often do you struggle with disappointment over how your life has turned out?

1	2	3	4	5	6	7	8	9	10
Daily				Sometimes					Never

9. How often do you struggle with feelings of envy or jealousy toward others?

1	2	3	4	5	6	7	8	9	10
Daily				Sometimes					Never

10. How well does your present reality measure up to what you expected life to be?

1	2	3	4	5	6	7	8	9	10
Falls short				About right					Far exceeds

RESULTS

10 – 30 = You are an extremely discontent person.

31 – 50 = You tend toward discontentment, probably because
you expect more than is realistic.

51 – 80 = You are a generally content person, able to take life
in stride.

80 – 100 = You should have written this book!

If your score fell into the first category, you may be a very unpleasant person to be around. You probably have trouble being satisfied, see the bad in every situation, and struggle with feelings of
bitterness. Reading this book may be a very important first step in
your journey toward a more healthy perspective on life.

If you fell into the second category, you have a lot of company.
Many struggle with frequent feelings of discontentment. You long to
maintain a sense of fulfillment, but you easily fall into patterns of
comparison, disappointment, and disillusionment. We will be examining several important principles to help you rise above your circumstances to a new level of living.

If you ended up in category three, you probably already have a
generally healthy attitude about your life. You can accept your circumstances without too much difficulty. You probably wish things
were a bit better than they are, but you've learned to cope. My hope is
that you will discover the secret to fully mastering contentment and
being a model for others.

If you are one of those few who scored in the fourth category,
then you've already discovered the joy and freedom of content living.
You may find nothing new in the pages of this book. It might simply
articulate what you've already discovered in your own life pilgrimage.

You are one of those rare individuals who holds the keys that can free others from the bondage of discontentment.

Whatever your personal situation may be, there is something to glean from a deeper evaluation of what we tend to expect from life and how we can move beyond the common traps which lead to discontentment.

Getting Personal

Have you allowed your expectations to bring mostly positive or negative results in your life? Have they led to positive discontentment which motivates you toward improvement, or negative discontentment which pushes you toward disillusionment? How can you work to reinforce the former and avoid the latter?

NOTE

1. Joe Dominguez and Vicki Robin, *Your Money or Your Life* (New York: Viking Penguin, 1992), 9.

Chapter Two

MAKING OURSELVES POOR

It is right to be contented with what we have, never with what we are. James Mackintosh

I am old enough to qualify as one of the last members of the now infamous baby-boom generation, and young enough to be on the front end of the next major emerging wave of culture makers—the baby busters. The boomers have been identified as those born between 1946 and 1964, the busters as those born from 1965 through 1976. These two groups represent more than 120 million Americans, the vast majority of our adult population.

Much has been written about the baby-boom generation and its impact upon the economy, culture, politics, religion, and every other facet of society. A wave of similar analysis is appearing about the baby busters who, as those just now starting families and entering the workforce, will collectively define our future way of life. Although some of the conclusions drawn are suspect, overgeneralized, and sensationalized, grains of truth in the research help us understand why the younger generations seem less content than others, and what factors have contributed to our expectations.

We could summarize the collective experience of the baby-boom and baby-bust generations into one phrase: They have had more, and come to expect more, than any other group in our history.

If we rearrange the biblical adage "To whom much is given much shall be required" to reflect our current generation, it could read "Those who have been given much, expect much more." Describing the baby boomers, author Landon Jones says,

> It is . . . the biggest, richest, and best educated generation America has ever produced. The boom babies were born to be the best and the brightest. They were the first raised in the new suburbs, the first with new televisions, the first in the new high schools. They were twice as likely as their parents to go to college and three times as likely as their grandparents. . . . Blessed with the great expectations of affluence and education, the boom children were raised as a generation of idealism and hope.[1]

Jones's observations also reflect the experience of the younger baby busters. They were born into all the advantages of their older counterparts, and then some. They have been described as less patient and more fussy. Savvy marketers know that they must provide goods and services faster, better, and cheaper if they hope to tap this younger, more demanding market. As a result, business is more competitive than ever.

The baby-boom and baby-bust crowds have defined our way of life, both for the better and for the worse. We have more, but we also expect more. We are consumed with ourselves—and no one feels bad about it. We have become far more concerned with personal well-being than with the good of society. Community and discipline have been lost to the surge of individualism and gratification that have come to dominate modern living. As a result, a sense of entitlement has swept over us. Most of us expect to receive benefits from society—yet feel no responsibility to give back to it. We have become contributors to and victims of a narcissistic culture. Psychologist David Brandt observes,

> In the case of the Boom Generation, doting parents and high expectations joined with social forces to produce an adult population which expected uninterrupted gratification. . . . Narcissism as a cultural phenomenon is so commonplace that we scarcely notice it. . . . No one bats an eye when a friend extols the virtues of *Looking Out for Number One, Winning Through Intimidation, Being One's Own Best Friend.* These are not just book titles, they are the clichés of the era.

The American ideal of rugged individualism has been replaced by the apotheosis of self.[2]

If these descriptions represent reality, we face a unique challenge in our pursuit of happiness and contentment. It is far more difficult to satisfy the indulged than the destitute.

In times past, people knew what it meant to wait. Great-grandmother may have wanted a sewing machine for five to ten years before she got one. Today, by contrast, our desires tend to be more short-term. We want, buy, and want again within a span of days, not years. By waiting, our ancestors *disciplined* their wants. By indulging our wants, we *intensify* them.

World-renowned psychologist Abraham Maslow summarized our struggle by describing the cycle of human needs and desires as a perpetual and constant progression. He said that we rarely reach a state of complete satisfaction in life except for a short time because . . .

> As one desire is satisfied, another pops up to take its place. When this is satisfied, still another comes into the foreground, and so on. It is a characteristic of human beings throughout their whole lives that they are practically always desiring something.[3]

Maslow described our motivation toward a better life as the pursuit of basic needs which fall into an ascending hierarchy. The most basic needs on the scale are the physiological or biological, such as air, food, or water. Once they have been met, we seek fulfillment of other needs, such as safety, belonging, love, self-esteem, and so on. Once we've attained a measure of each, we seek something better. In short, we never stop the pursuit of satisfaction because once one level has been attained, we raise the standard. Thus, the pattern of our generation is consistent with the pattern of human motivation.

In light of these dynamics, are we doomed to a life of disappointment and discontentment? Can we find the balance between greed and apathy, indulgence and lack?

I believe an important first step is to examine what we want from life. We can only understand our dissatisfaction when we understand our expectations. Right or wrong, good or bad, the things we expect from life have a major impact on our level of happiness.

WHAT WE EXPECT

It is difficult to accurately identify what we expect from life. Individual expectations vary from person to person and change from year to year. Expectations change with the seasons and circumstances of life.

Still, we can identify some of the broad categories of common wants. Whether or not we consciously acknowledge them, the majority of us share certain needs and desires.

Basic Provision

Regardless of status, everyone expects to have food, clothing, and a place to call home. Human history is filled with violent illustrations of what happens when these basic needs go unmet. When people are denied the opportunity to acquire them, they will revolt. They will turn against their leaders and steal from their friends. Otherwise peaceful people will become violent, if necessary, to feed their hungry children. We not only expect basic provisions, we demand them.

There was a time in the western world, not too long ago, when people devoted most of their energies to meeting these three primary needs—food, clothing, and shelter. Today, by contrast, we take them for granted. Even the poorest members of our society have some form of each—or could have them if they were willing to ask.

We come home from a fully-stocked supermarket and pay little attention to images on our television screens of hungry children. We not only cannot identify with their plight, it is beyond our comprehension how anyone could be in such want. Only a small portion of our senior population ever experienced similar struggles during the depression, but even for them it is a distant memory. We have moved beyond the days when basic provisions were the primary focus. That is good. But our bounty has left many of us complacent.

Material Possessions

I grew up in a typical middle-class home during the "wonder years" of the sixties and seventies. My home was stocked with the standard goods for the day—nice furniture, kitchen appliances, a station wagon in the garage, "hi-fi" stereo equipment, and, of course, a television set. We even had one of those new hand-held calculators! There were always presents under the tree at Christmas, and we wore the latest styles to school each year. We had most of the things anyone could want at the time.

I now have my own home. My wife and I could also be classified as the typical middle-class couple. We have most of the things my parents provided when I was a child, and then some. For example, we have a microwave oven in addition to the other kitchen appliances. (How did we survive without microwaves?) We have a CD player rather than a "hi-fi" turntable. (Record albums were so cumbersome!) Our television has a remote control. (We wouldn't want any unnecessary bodily motion.) And we have a VCR player. (Why limit ourselves to the shows provided by the networks?) We even have a home computer, something we never imagined would hit the average household when I was a boy. We have most of the material things we could want—at least until the latest and greatest comes along.

I have more belongings than my father, he had more than his father, and so on. My sons will probably have items in their homes that I can't even imagine today. That's the way it is supposed to be, right? We produce more stuff, want more stuff, and acquire more stuff. Material possessions are one of the primary ways that we rate our standard of living. We expect to have what our parents gave us, plus a little extra for good measure. In short, we expect to have possessions—lots of possessions!

Physical Health

Medical advances during this century have outpaced the wildest hopes of prior generations. We no longer expect to lose our sons and daughters to childhood diseases. Vaccinations have virtually eliminated most of these former killers. We no longer watch our loved ones die from mysterious infections. We simply pick up a prescription from the local drugstore. We have replaced home remedies with over-the-counter medication; superstitious rituals with corrective treatment; and chronic pain with Bayer, Tylenol, or Motrin. We are healthier and more quickly cured than any generation in history.

We have become so accustomed to health, however, that we seem more frightened by sickness. We no longer view it as part of

life, but as the ultimate enemy. Illness reminds us of our mortality—
something we don't want to face. We become visibly uncomfortable
around those who are seriously ill. Sickness is not supposed to inter-
rupt our lives—let alone take them from us. Physical health is not
just wanted, it is expected.

Financial Security

Pension plans, Social Security, retirement savings—all of these
represent a significant trend in our society. We want some form of
financial security to ensure a comfortable lifestyle today and tomorrow. But these common instruments were virtually unknown to earlier generations. Employers were not considered to be responsible to
plan for individuals' futures. Neither was the government. The individual and his or her family carried the burden of financial security.
The future was only as secure as a person's ability to work, but during tough times, others gave a helping hand.

When Roosevelt's New Deal brought in the social safety net, for
the first time in history, the government took responsibility for a nation in crisis to take care of large-scale poverty and starvation. By
design that responsibility was supposed to return to individuals when
the crisis ended. Unfortunately, it was never taken back. We still look
to government to ensure our future. As a result, we've stopped worrying about financial security and started expecting it.

Family Harmony

Belonging, love, affection, security, acceptance, encouragement,
instruction, companionship, laughter—they all find their best expression in the home. Few who are honest with themselves deny their
desire for a happy family life. We seek advice on finding a mate,
keeping the flame alive, building our child's self-esteem, relating to
grown kids, and grandparenting with grace. We want to land the perfect partner and live happily ever after. We want children who become best friends and grandchildren who sit on our laps. In short,
we want family harmony.

Our family expectations go beyond today and tomorrow, however. They also include yesterday. We want warm memories of Mom
in her apron baking cookies, Dad in the family room reading to

brother, and sister offering to help us with our homework. We compare our upbringing to the Walton or Brady family. If our experience was anything less, we accuse our parents of neglect, label our family dysfunctional, and mourn our lost childhood. We trace our negative emotions to parental failure and our dissatisfaction to unmet childhood needs. All of us want what none of us had—perfect parents and the ideal home. Many of us struggle with haunting memories of homes far from perfect. But no matter how hard we try, we cannot modify our memories to fit in the boxes we'd like them to fit.

There is a void in Carol's heart. She has spent her entire life trying to win the approval of her parents, to make them proud of her. They were good parents, sacrificing a great deal to provide her with a comfortable, secure home during her formative years. Now, as an adult, Carol wants them to see that the sacrifice was worthwhile.

Growing up in a large family made it difficult to get the attention Carol craved. She was the most compliant of five children, so her parents trusted her more than the others. There was rarely a need to discipline Carol, and she usually seemed quite happy and content. She was the ideal child, so she didn't take as much time and energy as the others.

During her high-school years, Carol was one of the most popular kids on campus. She was attractive and athletic, and she consistently made the dean's list for academic excellence. Carol was the type of student any parent would be proud of. Any parent, it seemed, except her own. They barely paid attention to her achievements. Oh sure, they loved her. But they were so busy dealing with the more needy kids in the family that there wasn't enough time to attend her games or award ceremonies. They felt that Carol was a good kid with lots of friends, so she didn't require as much attention as the others.

As she entered adulthood, Carol yearned for signs of approval from her parents. To hear them say, "We are so proud of you, Carol" would have brought joy. To learn that they had bragged about her accomplishments to their friends would have filled her empty spirit. But they didn't. The other kids had so many problems, they had little time to think about the one child who was doing things right. So she continued, unaware that her drive to achieve was really an attempt to prove herself worthy.

As the years have passed, Carol has become very successful in life. She is happily married, running her own cottage industry, rearing two lovely children, and serving in various service roles through her church. She has become everything an aging mom or dad could hope for in a daughter. Any parent would be proud to call her their daughter. Carol still wonders why her parents don't seem to notice.

Opportunity

I have several good friends who came to America as immigrants—bringing with them little more than the clothes they wore. They took advantage of the possibilities in this country and have become very successful. Through the decades many people of many nationalities have made their way to our "land of opportunity" for chances to fulfill dreams that could not be realized in their homelands.

Everyone wants the chance to better themselves. We seek more than to merely exist. We want to increase our knowledge, move up the ladder, expand our influence, advance our cause, and build our wealth. But we don't want any handouts—we much prefer to achieve on our own. All we want is the opportunity to make something of our lives. In America, we have come to expect it.

Rights

As a citizen of the United States, I can live and work wherever I want, vote for whomever I wish, worship as I see fit, speak out on matters I consider important, and own private property and possessions. Much good has come from the premise that every individual has certain "inalienable rights" which cannot be legally violated.

Our view of personal rights, however, has also fostered a widespread entitlement mentality. This has led many of us to view difficulty, lack, or inconvenience as a violation of our rights.

Happiness

When I was a senior in high school, my sociology teacher posed a question for discussion: "What do you most want from life?" After a few minutes for reflection, she went around the room and gave each of us the opportunity to tell our fundamental life objective—something very few of us had examined for more than three minutes.

As she circled the room for feedback, most of the responses reflected variations on the family-and-career themes dominating the hopes and plans of upcoming high school graduates. Then the teacher told us her own life ambition: "The highest goal of my life, the thing I want more than any other, is to be happy. No matter what I do, or where I go, or who I am with, I want happiness."

We were awestruck! Why didn't any of us think of that? We simplistically rambled on about college choices, family plans, and career hopes, but never gave thought to such a profound issue as our happiness. How could we be so shallow?

That teacher stated the dominant expectation of our generation. Like her, we want happiness above all else. We may not have it well defined, or have a plan for achieving it, but we know that we want it. And when we don't have it, we experience severe disappointment. Unfortunately, we fail to understand that happiness is a by-product, not a target. It comes when the other areas of our lives are properly aligned—especially our attitudes and objectives.

Looking back, perhaps it was the teacher who was shallow, and we students who had the right idea. I often wonder if she ever reached her goal. Perhaps, like many in our generation, she is still striving to attain an ill-defined yet passionately desired happiness.

Basic provisions, material possessions, physical health, financial security, family harmony, opportunity, rights, happiness—these are just some of the things we expect from life. None of them is necessarily bad. In fact, most of them are very good. Any expectation, if taken to an extreme, will lead to unhealthy attitudes in life. And the first step toward balance is to identify the sources of our dissatisfaction and the dynamics which may set us up to let us down.

STANDARD OF LIVING

Take a moment to think about your life. Evaluate the things you own, the people you love, the activities you enjoy, the work you do, the money you have, and the decisions you face. Contemplate the good and the bad, your successes and your failures, your blessings and your problems. Take a serious look at the whole package. Now answer this: Do you know anyone who has a better life than you?

Most of us confront this question in one form or another every day of our lives. We see how others live and compare their experiences to our own. Sometimes we look at those less fortunate and feel better about our circumstances, and other times we compare ourselves to those who are much better off—making ourselves jealous in the process. Either way, there is a fundamental flaw in our assessment. You see, no two people judge their satisfaction by the same criteria. Each of us has a unique "standard of living" by which we evaluate life. Therefore, it is impossible to know whether another person's life is better or worse than your own, because you do not know the person's basis of comparison. His standard may be far higher or lower than yours. He may be completely happy despite having less, or totally miserable despite having more. The critical ingredient is not what a person possesses in life, but rather what he expects from it. The same is true of us all. Therefore, it is important that we understand the factors which contribute to our own expectations—rather than measure our lives against someone else's standard.

STANDARD OF POVERTY

During my second year of college I had the opportunity to participate in a four-week trip to Korea as part of a short-term missions program. I had never traveled outside the United States and had no idea what to expect. The only words of wisdom I received from those who had gone on earlier trips was to fill my suitcase with packaged American foods as an alternative to the native cuisine.

We flew on one of the most modern, plush, efficient airliners of the day. In other words, there was no legroom for anyone over five feet tall, the restrooms were constantly occupied, and the meals tasted like the plastic containers in which they came. By the time the seventeen-hour trip was over, most of us were cranky, on edge, and ready to scream. The last thing I wanted to face as I exited the plane was a smiling, upbeat flight attendant telling me to have a nice day. Nothing could salvage the day ahead of me after the misery I'd been put through on that trip!

After a long drive to the outskirts of Seoul, we finally arrived at the home of a missionary family with whom we would be staying. They had a very nice home, much like the one I lived in back in the

States. They served us a good American meal, and we went to sleep in comfortable beds. Things were looking up.

We spent the following day walking through the city. I was not prepared for what I saw. Having spent my entire young life in the American middle class, I had no concept of how people in the third world lived. There were no neighborhood streets lined with two-story, colonial homes. They lived in row after row of frail, dirt-floor huts. There were no kids playing ball on neatly trimmed lawns with picket fences. Children were too busy working in the fields to spend time at play. There were no refrigerators filled with fresh food. Families were lucky to scrape together one meal at a time. They had no luxuries, lacked most of the material goods common to my home, and had few of life's "basic necessities." From my perspective, they lived in utter poverty. For some strange reason, however, they didn't seem to notice. They made the most of what they had, oblivious to how much they lacked.

I felt an overwhelming sense of shame for the attitudes I had demonstrated during the previous twenty-four hours. I complained about sub-standard food on the plane. They would have considered that same plate of food a feast fit for a king. I became irritated with the lack of comfort and cramped space on an otherwise enjoyable flight; walking was the highest form of transportation most of these people would ever experience. I had packed a suitcase full of snacks to avoid eating what they rationed for daily survival. My standard of sacrifice was their standard of wealth.

Why is it that one group of people can find fulfillment in the midst of surroundings which another person would find intolerable? Why was my standard of acceptable circumstances so much higher than theirs? After all, we both shared a common human spirit with an equal capacity for enjoying the good things of life. Why did I expect so much and they so little?

These questions can be applied without traveling to a third-world nation. The same dynamic occurs among the citizens of this generally affluent country. Men like Peter Lynch and Lee Iacocca have and expect a far higher standard of living than I will ever achieve. At the same time, I enjoy a lifestyle far beyond that of many within my own city. The wealthy among us consider middle-class living sub-standard, while the poor among us hope to someday achieve that same lifestyle.

This leads us to a key question. Why do we expect what we expect? Our expectations touch every aspect of our existence and establish the minimum acceptable standards for our fulfillment. If life fails to satisfy the approved criteria, happiness is put on hold.

Although we may not formally draft a checklist of expectations against which we intentionally measure our lives, each of us does have a list. It is written deep within our hearts, dictating our satisfaction with and response to the circumstances of life. It defines the content of our dreams and the "standard of living" we are willing to accept.

YOUR STANDARD

When you were born, you had no idea what to expect from life. Upon leaving the warmth and security of your mother's womb, you immediately encountered some pretty rough treatment. They slapped your bottom, cut your supply cord, stuck a suction device down your throat, and placed your shivering body under a stainless-steel bun warmer. If the first ten minutes were any indication of things to come, you could expect that postnatal life would be far from pleasant.

Things quickly improved. You discovered the joys of maternal love, the comfort of cotton blankets, and the relief of a good spit-up. Before long, your world expanded and your expectations enlarged. The more you experienced in life, the more you wanted from it. First a bottle, then a breadstick, then a burger. First a teddy bear, then a Tonka truck, then a Thunderbird. The more you saw and the more you sampled, the more you wanted.

By the time you reached adulthood, your expectations were firmly established. Various factors contributed to your list along the way. The way your family treated you contributed to how you expect to be treated by others. The types of food you ate as a child helped form your tastes as an adult. The house in which you lived set the standard for the one you hope to provide your own family.

Countless individual factors contribute to our differing expectations, and childhood experiences are only the beginning. What we read, what we are taught, our individual personality bent, the influence of friends, and a thousand other variables can impact our view of how life should be. Understanding those variables can help us identify why we expect what we expect.

Natural Desires

God designed each of us with the desire for certain things in life. These passions are natural, healthy, and an essential part of our make-up. They range from physical hunger to the search for meaningful relationships and personal significance. These desires impact our attitudes and motivate our actions toward every circumstance and opportunity we face. Properly focused, they also point the human family in the direction intended by our Creator.

I work with a forty-year-old single man who has a strong desire to marry. He wants long-term companionship, physical intimacy, children, and all the things that go along with marriage. Yet, for some reason, he feels guilty about the intensity of his desire. He feels that if he were a more mature Christian, his relationship to God would satisfy all such longings. Rather than view his desire for a mate as a natural outgrowth of his humanity, he sees it as a sign of his carnality. But he is mistaken.

We often condemn ourselves over our innate desires, rather than viewing them as a natural part of God's wonderful design. It is OK to desire the companionship and intimacy of a loving husband or wife. It is not selfish to want children, a healthy body, a better job, or the acceptance of others. These desires do not necessarily reveal a lack of faith in God, a poor self-image, or a selfish disposition. They could simply reveal that you have a serious case of humanity. Just as it was foolish when I was a teenager to ask God to take away my attraction to girls, it is foolish to chastise ourselves over the natural desires He built into our design. The desire for things such as comfort, companionship, significance, and posterity are part of our make-up and foundational needs which contribute to our list of life expectations.

Upbringing

Regardless of how good or bad your childhood may have been, it had a tremendous impact on what you expect from life today. It is virtually impossible to separate what you experienced yesterday from what you hope to experience tomorrow. If you were reared in a wealthy home, you may find it difficult to step down to middle-class living. If your parents made you feel like a prince or princess, you will likely expect the same from your mate today. On the other end of the spectrum, those who experienced abuse or neglect as children often find themselves accepting similar treatment in adulthood. Many are drawn into such relationships despite early warning signs of abuse and disrespect—never seriously questioning the pattern because it is consistent with early experiences which conditioned them to expect no better.

I have been concerned over our growing tendency to lay the blame for every wrong act or attitude at the feet of our parents. This trend has led us down the path of blame-shifting when we fail and parent-bashing when we hurt. We must avoid the obvious extremes that can come when we overscrutinize our upbringing. At the same time, however, we cannot minimize the impact of parental influence on our lives. All of us enter adulthood with the deeply-ingrained imprint of childhood experiences. Those experiences have a tremendous influence over how we view what life should be.

I was one of seven children. As you can imagine, there was little time and less patience for whining in such a large family. If I hurt myself while playing, and it wasn't serious, Mom would provide an obligatory five-second hug and send me on my way. Long, drawn-out sympathy sessions were out of the question. After all, there were seven clumsy kids in our house and no time for excessive pampering. Thus, I grew up expecting the world to respond to my hurts with a cordial pat on the back before sending me on my way. As an adult, I respond to discouragement and pain differently than those who received a high degree of empathy and solace in response to minor childhood pains. Today, I tend to minimize the significance of my emotional pain, while others may become so introspective that they never move beyond it.

If a child was smart, he never expressed boredom or self-pity within earshot of my parents. Instead of the desired sympathy, he could quickly be assigned chores to help forget his misery. Hard work was seen as the best medicine for getting one's mind off himself. As my parents would say, the happiest people in the world are those too busy to feel sorry for themselves. By contrast, many were raised in families in which Mom and Dad responded to momentary gloom or doldrums with sympathetic indulgence. On the up side, these folks turn out to be a great support when you need a shoulder to cry on. On the down side, they can also expect to be rescued from the valleys of life rather than work through them.

Countless subtle dynamics help shape our outlook on life. Though the specifics vary, the principle is the same in all of our lives. Childhood experiences and upbringing have a dramatic impact upon what we expect from life and how we react to it.

Religious Teachings

Jeff expected his life to turn out better than it has. Despite an intense desire to marry, he's still single at forty. He is concerned that the majority of his opportunities may be behind him. He is stuck in a dead-end job, having been overlooked for promotion on several occasions. He drives an old, rusty Ford that leaves oil stains on the concrete wherever he parks. He has little money, much debt, and virtually no social life. Life is nothing like he expected.

Shortly after becoming a Christian during his early adult years, Jeff became part of a group that taught him God would fulfill all the desires of his heart. If he dedicated his life to the Lord's service, so they said, his needs would be met and his hopes realized. In Jeff's mind, their general teaching translated into very specific expectations. He trusted God to provide him with a wife—preferably an attractive, fun-loving one. He took a low-paying job with a parachurch ministry, counting on the Lord to meet all his financial needs as part of the deal. After all, they told him that God would come through if Jeff was willing to yield all. Jeff did, but it seems as though God didn't. Now he struggles with bitterness and anger. Life didn't turn out as it was supposed to, and it is because God didn't hold up His end of the bargain.

Jeff is typical of many Christians who have built their life expectations around religious instruction. They were taught to trust God for this or wait on the Lord for that, and they never questioned whether or not the formula was based upon biblical truth. As a result, they put themselves in a position of facing ongoing unmet expectations and spiritual disillusionment. Some are taught that the Christian life should be free of sickness and pain if they have enough faith. Others learn that God is a cosmic killjoy waiting to pounce on them if they have any fun. Still others spend life waiting for a miracle to rescue them from their difficulties. Regardless of the specifics, the problem is the same. We expect from God what He may never have promised. We add items to our list of life expectations in response to the things we are taught—often setting ourselves up for a fall in the process.

Media Images

Ours is the first generation in history which has been dominated by a media industry. Movies, magazines, network and cable television programs, advertisements, radio talk shows, music videos, books, on-line computer networks, and more influence our expectations from life. Like a ringing bell to Pavlov's dogs, their images generate the intended response in us, their willing victims. They tell us what we don't have and how to get it. They tell us we aren't rich enough, smart enough, attractive enough, healthy enough, or popular enough. We bombard our minds with the images they portray, and then wonder why we struggle with contentment in life.

Associations

It has been said that you are what you read and who you spend time with. In other words, the ideas you ponder and the people you associate with have a tremendous influence upon the person you will become. The same principle is true with regard to the things we desire from life. In fact, I am convinced that our associations have a stronger impact upon our expectations than the media images around us.

My wife and I were married just before our last year of college. With normal living expenses and tuition payments to manage, we had very little money or material possessions. We rented a government-subsidized apartment, drove an old car, and dined on a folding card table. Most of our friends were in the same situation, so we didn't mind.

Following graduation, my wife began her teaching career and I entered graduate school. We were committed to getting me through my masters program without debt, so we applied her income toward tuition and books. My income, meager as it was, dictated our lifestyle. Obviously, we stayed in the low-rent apartment and continued driving the old car and eating off the folding card table. This arrangement went on for several years, and it started bothering us. Nothing had changed in our lifestyle from a few years earlier, except our ·friends. Most of them were finished with school and on to a different stage of life. They were buying new homes, driving nice cars, and enjoying meals on real dining-room furniture. The more time we spent with our friends, the less content we became with our own living situation. The less time we spent with friends, the more we enjoyed the little we had. The fact that we were poor only bothered us when our friends became comparatively rich. Thus, our associations had a tremendous impact upon our level of contentment.

I do not recommend that you dump any friends or avoid those family members who have more than you do. I am simply suggesting that your associations will affect what you expect from life. When your best friend buys a new car it hits you harder than any television advertisement. If your younger sister has a baby while you struggle to get pregnant, it will bother you more than every Shirley Temple movie combined. Personal associations have a significant impact upon what we expect from life and our effort to remain content.

Natural desires, upbringing, religious teachings, media images, and our associations are only a few of the many factors which contribute to our list of life expectations. We could also examine the subtle impact of cultural values, personal security needs, the drive for acceptance, sibling competition, and countless other issues which directly and indirectly form the context of our desires. The particulars vary from individual to individual and lay the foundation for what we seek and pursue from life. We are disappointed when their promises remain unfulfilled.

In addition to our individual standards, societal trends can have a tremendous impact upon our expectations. We cannot separate our personal expectations from the economic and social context in which our lives unfold, and it is wise to explore the impact they have upon our view of how life should be.

THE BEST AND WORST OF TIMES

I recall fondly my early relationship with my grandparents. They periodically told us details of the way things were when they were children. You know the stories—walking miles to school in the cold, receiving nothing but an orange in the stocking on Christmas morning and being grateful for it! As a comparatively spoiled youngster, I couldn't fully appreciate the lifestyle contrast they described. But the details of their legacy have stuck with me as a reminder that life has not always been so good.

My grandparents lived through one of the most difficult periods in American history—The Great Depression. They learned the meaning of going without and how to find happiness apart from material possessions, of which they had few. With rare exception, everyone was going through an equally tough time during the decade of the 1930s. Few encountered prosperity, and none were untouched by the economic devastation around them. Parents feared the possibility that they would lose the ability to provide for their children. Few bought the government's rhetoric about prosperity being right around the corner. Times were tough and were expected to stay that way for some time.

Despite the best efforts of a progressive government, the only thing able to pull the nation out of decline was an equally unpleasant alternative, war. Our boys entered, and won, the fight against tyranny in Europe and Asia. America traded the forced sacrifices of economic collapse for the voluntary sacrifices of helping soldiers defeat Hitler and company. They did, and to the victor went the spoils. The painful memories of a devastating war were eased by the phenomenal economic prosperity which followed.

Happy Days

Economic stagnation and decline suddenly turned to opportunity and growth. Jobs became plentiful, the suburbs flourished with newly-formed young families, and the pursuit of the American dream was underway. People were making up for lost time. It was time to reap the rewards of the simultaneous victory over poverty and the Third Reich.

In this context a new generation was born. America entered a period which would later be dubbed the baby-boom years. Maternity wards were overwhelmed by the sudden increase in birthrates across the country. Young couples were free, wealthy, and optimistic. There was no better time to start a family—and millions did just that.

More than four million children were born each year during this golden era. Few of them knew anything of the intense sacrifices their parents had experienced during the prior two decades. How could they understand such poverty in the midst of such affluence? Postwar parents worked hard to give their kids a better childhood than they had had to endure. Their era of sacrifice was over, and they weren't going back.

A Culture of Optimism

Year after year, our standard of living has continued to improve. We build bigger homes, drive flashier cars, attend better schools, and wear more stylish clothes. The past few decades have seen us go from radio, to stereo, to black-and-white television, to big-screen home-entertainment systems. Every aspect of life seemed to be on a track toward better and better. As a result, we have become a culture of optimism, each generation expecting to exceed the previous in living standards. We've developed and embraced a fundamental American birthright—upward mobility.

It would be difficult to overestimate the impact prosperity has had upon our cultural expectations. Americans are an optimistic people. We view ourselves as the best and the brightest, the king of the hill, the envy of the world. We expect to win, to prosper, to be first, to be best, and to have it all. We truly believe that anything is possible, and we turn those who accomplish great things into national heros and media celebrities.

We like winners, not losers. Only recently have we overcome the national shame and skepticism caused by our experience with Vietnam. We couldn't handle a loss on our record, and it took a Desert Storm victory to regain our self-respect. I remember well the euphoria generated by the news that we had quickly and decisively defeated the Iraqi army. We were back on top, and we could rightfully reclaim our lost sense of national pride.

The largest segment of our current adult population was born into a culture of affluence. As a result, we have come to expect prosperity and opportunity. Unfortunately, our optimism may become the basis of our disappointment.

51

Downward Mobility

John and Linda are a young couple in their late twenties. They met and fell in love during college, just like their parents. They were married shortly after graduation, just like their parents. They hope to achieve the American dream, just like their parents.

John and Linda both work long hours to make ends meet, unlike their parents. They live in a small apartment because they can't afford to buy a house of their own, unlike their parents. They fully expect to place any future children into day-care because it seems to them that wives can no longer afford the luxury of staying home with the kids, unlike their parents. Despite graduating with honors from college, John found it necessary to accept a service industry job that pays little more than minimum wage, about the same as Linda's administrative assistant role. It seems that an education no longer guarantees career advancement, like it did for their parents. John and Linda are fairly happy, but they wonder whether or not they will ever achieve their goals or reach the standard of living they had expected.

John and Linda are typical of many baby-bust and younger baby-boom couples. They have the same aspirations as their parents and grandparents, but they seem to have less opportunity. The government takes more of their paycheck, and there are fewer high-paying jobs—even for college graduates—requiring two incomes just to reach the standard of living Dad achieved with his nine-to-five factory job. For several complex cultural reasons, an emerging generation of American adults may never attain the lifestyle they experienced as children—let alone exceed it.

Postwar parents may have been better prepared to enjoy the good things of life than their children who have always had them. Going without set them up for the pleasure of having it all. Having it all set their children up for the disappointment of going without.

Spoiled by Prosperity

My wife and I have spent the past eight years ministering among newly married couples—most of which have been married three years or less. During one discussion session, I posed several questions regarding their most common fears entering family life together.

One of those questions related to standard of living. It was interesting to discover that virtually every couple expressed the same concern. They feared the very real probability that they would never live as well as their parents. If they wanted a nice suburban home, they would need two incomes. If they wanted the wife to become a full-time homemaker when kids came along, they would need to live in a less desirable part of town, drive an old car, and forget about new furniture. Other specifics were raised, all pointing to the same reality. They would need to lower the lifestyle standards they had been conditioned from childhood to expect.

Cutting a few corners and sacrificing a few luxuries is no major catastrophe—particularly in a country where the poor among us have more than the wealthy of other lands. The issue is not how bad our living standard has become, but rather how difficult it is to accept less than we expected. Perpetual success and prosperity conditioned us to view upward mobility as a national birthright. Now that the trend seems to be changing, how will we deal with the resulting disappointment?

It is far more difficult to sacrifice something you've already experienced and come to expect than something you've not yet attained. Ask anyone who has consciously decided to lower his lifestyle in order to get out of debt. It was relatively easy for my wife and me to live in a small low-rent apartment during our first four years of marriage because it was better than the crowded college dorms we had endured the prior four years. It would be difficult now, however, to return to that lifestyle after living in a nice home with a yard. In the same way, it is more difficult for today's younger generations to accept a lower standard of living than their parents because they have grown accustomed to the comforts and luxuries. After being spoiled by the good life, many of us are facing the realities of sacrificing some of our wants for the first time—and we don't like it.

Getting Personal . . . .

How have the general trends and changes in society shaped your expectations? How do these expectations dictate your satisfaction with the circumstances of life? Take a few moments to contemplate what factors have influenced your personal "standard of living."

NOTES

1. Landon Y. Jones, *Great Expectations* (New York: McCanne Geoghegan, 1980), 1.
2. David Brandt, *Is That All There Is?* (New York: Poseidon Press, 1984), 103–4.
3. Abraham H. Maslow, *Motivation and Personality,* 3d ed. (New York: Harper & Row, 1987), 7.

Chapter Three

THE MYTH OF HAPPILY EVER AFTER

Too many people miss the silver lining because they're expecting gold. Maurice Seitter

H ave you ever noticed that promotional brochures always seem to show things better than they actually are? Vacation spots are always warm and sunny, hotels are always plush, and Big Macs never look squashed. Why is that?

Brochures always represent things in the best possible light, and they never show the bad points. They exaggerate at best, and lie at worst. This lesson applies to more than vacation spots or fast-food burgers. It is true of everything in life. We create a "brochure" with our expectations—the things we wish for, hope for, and work for. We paint a picture in our hearts of how our lives should be, and we describe the future in the best possible light. We exaggerate the possibilities at best, and outright lie to ourselves at worst. Unfortunately, life rarely turns out to be like the brochure.

The stories we grew up on weren't much more true to our everyday experience. "Once upon a time" always ended with "and they lived happily ever after." Unfortunately, it usually doesn't work that way. In fact, I am convinced that "happily ever after" is nothing but a myth.

Have you ever wondered what actually happened to Cinderella after her foot fit the glass slipper? What about Sleeping Beauty? Did everything turn out well for her and Prince Charming? And let's not forget Snow White. We know that she survived the poison apple thanks to a kiss from the handsome prince, but how did she and the seven dwarfs make out afterward? I want to know specific details. What was everyday life like for these characters much later, after Walt Disney lost interest?

Let's check in on Cinderella years after the glass slipper incident. As you may recall, she went to the palace and married the prince—finally free from the demands of her wicked stepmother and stepsisters. What you may not know is that her new mother-in-law, the queen, turned out to be a royal pain in the neck. She resented Cinderella for stealing her son's affections, and she let it be known in many ways. The palace was never clean enough for her, and she constantly complained that Cinderella didn't feed the prince as well as when he was at home. Of course, the children only misbehaved in front of their grandmother, leading her to criticize Cinderella's maternal abilities. To make matters worse, the prince always seemed to take his mother's side. Cinderella felt unappreciated in her role as homemaker. She eventually gave up trying and now spends most days eating chocolate bonbons and reading fairy-tale books, comparing her miserable life to that lucky girl who married good-looking Prince Philip.

Speaking of Mrs. Prince Philip, Sleeping Beauty lives in a neighboring castle. How did things turn out for her? Beauty and Charming had a wonderful honeymoon, as you might expect of such an attractive and romantic couple. He was proud to have such a lovely wife, and she to have such a handsome husband. Each was smitten with the other's picture-perfect appearance. They were a match made in heaven, or so it seemed. But then, one day, something terrible happened. They began to age. Her baby-soft skin started to wrinkle and her perfect figure expanded. His wavy hair started falling out, and his muscular chest started falling down. Much to their horror, Beauty and Charming were starting to look like normal people! The basis of their love was eroding away, and they could do nothing to stop it. He lost interest in her, and she lost track of him. He spent more time at the office; she spent more money at the mall. They became strangers living in the same palace. The marriage eventually ended after he ran off with a younger beauty. Beauty got the castle in the divorce settlement—but it was little consolation in light of how her life turned out. She has become so anxious over the whole ordeal that she needs prescription sleeping pills to get any rest at all.

Snow White ended up with serious problems of her own. She and her prince settled down in a little mansion not far from the home of the seven dwarfs. It's a good thing too. The dwarfs had to come to Snow's aid after her husband's nervous breakdown. It seems he couldn't handle her compulsive whistling whenever she worked around the house. That happy, joyful spirit of hers was very appealing during courtship. But it drove him nuts several years into the marriage. After he was admitted to the asylum, she went back to work for the dwarfs—cleaning their laundry and cooking their meals.

See what I mean? "Happily ever after" isn't all that it's cracked up to be. Even the most perfect lives run into problems now and then.

DEBUNKING THE MYTH

Most of us look forward to some event, status, person, or experience to move our lives beyond "once upon a time" toward "happily ever after." Perhaps we expect to ride off into the sunset with our handsome prince or beautiful princess to live in eternal bliss. For some it may be the desire for a certain status or salary at work. Others may want a wicked stepmother, or some other undesirable person, to permanently exit their life. Regardless of the specific longing, the impact is the same. We cannot find contentment with life as it is because we're eagerly waiting for our happy ending to come.

Sooner or later, however, we must all accept the reality that "happily ever after" will never arrive. Even if the promotion comes, there will be new sources of frustration on the job. Even if you get the raise, it will not be enough money. Even if the wedding day arrives, he or she will not meet your every need. Even if you get rid of that problem person, another will come behind him. No matter what the dream, it cannot bring you into a state of permanent tranquillity and happiness.

Have you ever daydreamed about winning a sweepstakes? Imagine having no more worries about overdue bills, building a brand-new house to replace the one with a leaky roof, driving a new sports car instead of the rusty four-door with balding tires. The more noble among us imagine giving a large sum of money to our church or favorite charity—making us feel better about the personal-indulgence binge we plan to pursue once our numbers pay off. And yet, would winning large sums of money really solve all our problems and bring us to a new level of living?

Actually, it could solve some of our problems, particularly if we have overdue bills and grand financial goals. However, instant wealth also brings with it a whole new set of struggles—many of which are far more serious than those left behind. The stories are all too common. A once happy family becomes a broken home a few years after winning millions. A man who dreamed of what winning the lottery could do for him regrets what it has done to him. A relatively unknown person becomes an instant star—especially to those who want a piece of the pie. Sweepstakes and lotteries, expected to bring the good life to the winner, often bring a measure of the bad life with them. For whatever reasons, instant wealth often brings instant trouble.

The same is true for those who think marriage will fill the void of loneliness in their lives. Quite often, those who most desperately desire a mate to bring them happiness are those least able to make a marriage work. Even the most sensitive man in the world cannot meet every need his wife has. Nor can the most supportive wife fulfill her husband's every desire. Those who enter a relationship hoping for "happily ever after" often learn this lesson the hard way.

The hard truth is this: No person, event, status, experience, or accomplishment will bring us into a state of permanent happiness. Fulfilled dreams may bring short-term pleasure or even temporary meaning to our lives. But they cannot bring us to the place of contentment we seek. If contentment is not found and fostered without them, it will not come with them. "Happily ever after" is a myth. Until we are willing to accept that reality, fulfillment in life will remain a distant fairy tale.

REAL LIFE

Changing diapers, paying bills, cleaning laundry, punching a clock, mowing the lawn, washing dishes, bathing kids, dusting furniture, waiting in lines, driving in traffic, rotating the tires, and repairing the sink. These are the daily realities of modern life. They are the sum of our days—and the source of our disappointment. Somehow, we expected something better.

Jennifer grew up in a typical middle-class home in the Midwest. She had one brother, two loving parents, and a color television set. She never missed a meal, always dressed nice, and had most of the latest toys. Jennifer attended a modern public school where she received academic instruction and a wonderful church where she received spiritual training.

During her adolescent years, Jennifer faced some tough times. She experienced the humiliation of acne, the awkwardness of lanky, and the confusion of puberty. But her loving parents were always there at the right moment to bolster her waning self-esteem. She made it through just fine, growing into a lovely young lady.

Jennifer learned many valuable lessons growing up. The television taught her that she could expect to live happily ever after, the stories in Sunday school taught her that God would bless her if she lived a good life, and her parents taught her that she was the most special person on earth. She grew up with a fit body, sharp mind, strong faith, and high self-esteem. Jennifer was ready for a good life.

During college, Jennifer met a wonderful man with whom she fell in love—just like in the movies. They married after graduation, landed great jobs, and purchased a nice home in the suburbs—just like on television. After a few years, Jennifer had a baby and decided to quit work and be a homemaker—just like Mom. The good Lord blessed Jennifer beyond measure—just like the Sunday school teachers had said He would.

Unfortunately, Jennifer isn't happy. She finds the daily routine of motherhood unfulfilling. She went back to work for more of a challenge, but missed her kids. She returned home to be a good mother, but craves adult conversation and lunch outings that don't include ketchup packets. Jennifer resents her husband's long hours at work. He isn't as romantic as he was during courtship, and she wonders whether or not he appreciates all her efforts. She has nothing to look forward to other than more dishes and diapers.

Many of us face the same dilemma Jennifer experienced. Even if somehow we get everything we wanted, we've discovered that everything we wanted isn't enough. We, like her, were set up for a fall by the lessons of modern life. Life as it is doesn't seem to be enough.

→We want more excitement, less monotony—more punch, less pinch. We hope for the day our life turns to "happily ever after." Unfortunately, that day rarely comes.

When Your Dream Doesn't Come True

Let's face it, all of us have some special dream we long to see fulfilled. For some the dream may be winning the lottery, for others meeting Mr. Right, or being handed a key to the executive washroom, or publishing a best-selling novel, or watching a son graduate with honors . . . from Harvard. The specifics vary from person to person, but the secret yearning is the same for all. We want something extraordinary to rescue us from the mediocrity of life.

The good news is that you may be one of those people who accomplish all of their goals and realize all of their dreams. The bad news is that you probably aren't. Only about one person in six billion has a life like that. And since you probably already know (and hate) someone who qualifies, your chances are rather slim.

Don't get me wrong; I'm no pessimist. In fact, I tend to see possibilities where others only see obstacles. But I've also come to accept the fact that circumstances do not always cooperate with our dreams. No matter how much I want or expect something to occur, God may have other plans for me. Those unable to cope with that reality are in for a rough ride.

Some time ago a television advertisement featured a young boy patiently waiting as his favorite brand of ketchup slowly poured from its bottle onto a naked hamburger. Because this ketchup was thick with flavor, the ad implied, it was well worth the anticipation. Watching the boy bite into the hamburger and lick his chops made a convincing case. The ad reinforced an important principle. When you are expecting something good, anticipation can be a delightful part of the process.

That is fine for a five-year-old at lunch. But what about those situations in which you wait, and wait, and wait some more, yet the good you expected never arrives? In those times, anticipation is a cruel substitute for satisfaction.

We have all known the frustration of hoping for the best, only to experience the worst. It is in these times that the excitement of anticipation sours into the stench of disillusionment. No one enjoys it. No one wants it. But in one way or another, we all live with it.

Fruitless Anticipation

Mark has been working the same factory job for more than twenty years. He has been overlooked for promotion on ten different occasions, but no other company is hiring people with his skills, and he doesn't want to start over in a different field. He feels trapped.

Robert and Mary wanted a big family—four, maybe five kids. After ten years of marriage, they still have empty arms. They have been to fertility specialists, leading to two pregnancies which ended in two miscarriages. They can't handle another heartbreaking disappointment.

James has known what he wanted to be since he was a little boy—a pilot. After he accepted Christ as a teenager, he decided he would be a missionary pilot. Six months ago he graduated from Bible college and began training for missionary aviation. He has just been diagnosed with diabetes, which disqualifies him to fly.

Now What?

Though their specific circumstances differ, Mark, Robert and Mary, and James are all encountering the same struggle. Each of them has confronted the possibility of never attaining his or her dreams. They've all asked the same important question . . . Now what?

How do you experience satisfaction in life when your deepest longings are unfulfilled? Can Mark know fulfillment even in a routine, dead-end job? Can Robert and Mary maintain a strong marriage in spite of their deep disappointments? Can James learn to trust God's plan for his life even though he feels right now that God has been cruel to his dreams and longings? The answer is simple: It all depends upon how they respond.

THE BEST-LAID PLANS

Our ability to cope with unmet expectations depends upon whether or not we can come to terms with life as it is, rather than life as we want it to be. Our plans, no matter how noble, do not dictate the circumstances of life. We must learn to adapt and accept unplanned circumstances.

Like many people, I usually list goals for the coming year on New Year's Day. I also take time at the end of each year to record some of the key events of the previous twelve months. I reflect on the high points, the low points, and some of the most meaningful moments. Guess what? The things I list on December 31 rarely match the plans I had recorded on January 1. Some turn out better than I had hoped. Some turn out worse. All of them turn out different.

Life is more like sailing than walking. When we walk, we are generally in control of our course. When sailing, on the other hand, we are at the mercy of changing weather or shifting winds. Despite our best efforts, variables beyond our control have a profound impact upon the direction and speed of our journey.

The Winds of Change

I am the type of person who plans his course and actively pursues one goal after another. When I was younger, I had little doubt as to what I would be doing five or ten years later. I knew where I would attend college, what type of career I would pursue, whom I would marry, and the timing of each step needed to attain my long-range goals.

Fifteen years later, my degree is from another school, I'm working in a different profession, and I am married to a person I hadn't even met yet. I see little similarity between my earlier plans and the real experiences of the past decade. The winds of life blew in a different direction. My confident assessment of the future was wrong, and I couldn't be happier.

I've learned a very important lesson while sailing the seas of life. I cannot control my circumstances. They will come as they come, whether I like it or not. They will change my course, and I can't do a thing about it. The choice is simple: I can choose to become bitter when they sink my plans, or I can pursue the new opportunities they offer. The second option makes the journey far more pleasant.

Unfortunately, I have encountered many people who consistently choose option one. They are unhappy because circumstances fail to cooperate with their dreams. They believe that life has handed them, and only them, a raw deal. Rather than question their expectations, however, they blame circumstances, people, society, and even God for their misery.

I have also known many individuals who refuse to sink into a cycle of blame and bitterness when reality falls short of their dreams. Some of the happiest people I have met are those who've learned to rise above the disappointment of unmet expectations, despite severe loss and hardship in life. They are an inspiration to me and a mystery to many.

Living for Someday

We often neglect the wisdom of James 4:13–15, which warns of presuming upon the future. It is foolish to hope that future events will rescue us from present unhappiness. Joy is a daily choice, not a future hope.

Our local newspaper includes a section highlighting little-known but official "holidays" of the coming week. I've seen such major events as "Poinsettia Day" and "Underdog Day." Of course, I do my best to celebrate each one of them. This week is very special indeed. You see, Tuesday is the official "Evaluate Your Life Day." Friday has been given equal billing as "World's End Day." In other words, I am supposed to evaluate my life on Tuesday before I lose it on Friday. What's the point?

Could it be that these symbolic days share the same week for a reason? After all, honestly facing the brevity of life helps put things in proper perspective.

Let's pretend that it is Tuesday, and you must evaluate your life in anticipation of Friday. Would you find that you've been holding out for a "someday" that may never come? Has your existence been anticipating joyful living rather than experiencing it? Are there certain events which must take place before you can be happy?

Most of us live anticipating someday, rather than enjoying today. We can hardly wait for graduation, and then for a good job, and then for promotion, and then for vacation, and then for retirement. We look forward to the day baby is out of diapers, and then to the day he is in school, and then to the day he finishes college, and then to the day he brings the grandkids for a visit. Won't it be great when . . . Things will improve after . . . Maybe someday we'll . . . And on and on it goes. We live for a better tomorrow, while letting today slip through our fingers.

There is nothing wrong with looking forward to future events. In fact, the pursuit of better things often motivates diligence and hard work as we seek to improve our lot in life. But there is a vast difference between drawing upon tomorrow's rewards for motivation and depending upon tomorrow's events for happiness.

If we base our happiness upon future events, then our happiness is uncertain. If, on the other hand, we can discover the secret to happiness apart from circumstances, we may find that we can experience a rewarding, fulfilling life whether or not our life matches our plans.

GREENER GRASS

We've heard it said that the grass is always greener on the other side of the fence. Yet, most of us spend our lives envying others, wishing we had their obviously better life circumstances. Well, I'll let you in on a little secret. The person you think has it made thinks someone else has it better. Who knows, it may even be your lot that the other person fancies.

Barb and Jill

Barb is a thirty-three-year-old single woman. She has a great career in advertising, drives a sporty car, and lives in an upscale apartment in the nicest part of town. She has been successful in her job, leads a singles group at her church, and spends her weekends enjoying the company of good friends. She has everything a professional girl could ever want—except happiness. In the midst of her busy lifestyle and many friends, Barb struggles with boredom and loneliness.

For as long as she can remember, Barb has wanted a family. She has dated several guys, but never fell for any of them. She respects herself too much to settle for second best. But she is getting concerned that she may end up with no one. She would give up her nice car, freedom, and accomplishments in a minute to have a life like her kid sister, Jill.

Jill is thirty years old, married to a nice fellow named Stan, and spends her days caring for several cute but rambunctious children.

Jill and Stan were married shortly after graduating from college. It wasn't long before they discovered they were expecting their first child. Jill put her career plans on hold because she was committed to being at home with her children—at least until they reached school-age. Jill and Stan agreed that the role of mother was more important than money, and keeping her at home would be worth the necessary sacrifices. Eight years and three children later, Jill is still a homemaker.

Jill has discovered that motherhood is a thankless job. She spends three hundred and sixty-five days a year caring for the needs of her children and husband, and all she gets in return is an annual Mother's Day card. She serves as household business manager, minor surgeon, family counselor, gourmet chef, cleaning service, academic tutor, and part-time chauffeur—yet receives no promotions or annual reviews to let her know whether or not she is appreciated. Jill often feels like an indentured servant to her family, longing for a bit of freedom. She would love to treat herself to a night on the town—the kind her big sister Barb often enjoys. Unfortunately, even if she had the time, she wouldn't have the money. Living on one income requires a very tight budget. She would love to buy herself cute clothes and drive a new car—like Barb. In fact, Jill thinks a life like her sister Barb's would be much better than a life spent cleaning dirty laundry and wiping runny noses.

Pastor Bill and Reverend Greg

Pastor Bill pastors a small, rural church of just over one hundred members. Everyone knows one another by name, and supporting one another comes as natural as breathing. Unlike many large-city congregations, Bill's church has a loving, family atmosphere. They even call one another brother and sister.

Of course, in addition to loving support for one another, siblings are also known for rivalry. And the brothers and sisters at Pastor Bill's church are no exception. They fight with one another, criticize one another, and talk behind one another's back—all in brotherly love. They expect perfection from Bill and his family, become jealous if he spends more time with one member than another, and get upset when he welcomes a visitor to the church. After all, he barely spends enough time with the people already in the church. Why in the world would he want any more in the flock than he already has?

Bill faces discouragement on a regular basis. He becomes weary with the petty conflict among members and the unreasonable expectations on his time. He often dreams of how great it would be to pastor a larger congregation where such problems were not so common—like Reverend Greg's church.

Reverend Greg indeed pastors a big church, one of the largest in his denomination. In fact, it recently went from two to three Sunday morning services just to accommodate the large crowds. If you measure success by size, as do many pastors, you'd consider Reverend Greg's church an overwhelming success.

But Greg measures success by a higher standard than mere growth, and he is not at all satisfied with what is happening at the church. In fact, he is concerned that rapid growth may be contributing to the church's downfall. The church is growing so quickly, the pastoral staff can't keep up. People with pastoral-care needs are beginning to feel neglected, new members are joining with little or no sense of commitment, every new person brings a new counseling demand, even the parking lot is too small for all the cars it must accommodate. Several board members recently suggested that the church launch a full-scale building program to keep pace with the growth, and everyone knows that the senior pastor must oversee the fund-raising effort. Reverend Greg is starting to feel more like a supervisor than a shepherd—trying to keep all this activity on schedule and on budget rather than attending to the needs of his flock.

Often, when the pressure becomes too much to bear, Greg longs for the days when he pastored a smaller church—where everyone knew one another by name and the biggest problems he had to deal with were petty conflicts and member expectations.

Bob and John

Bob is a software-design specialist for a large communications corporation. In other words, he sits in front of a computer screen all day writing line after line of code. Although the job pays a decent salary, it also drains the life out of him. He has virtually no interaction with people, very little opportunity for advancement because he deals with information rather than personnel, and no new challenge because he is assigned to the same project day in and day out. In short, Bob is bored to tears with his job. He would much prefer a position like John's, which involves many people and daily challenge.

John works with the same company as manager of the order-processing division. He has a staff of more than fifty, manages a budget of nearly one million dollars, and serves as project leader of seven business teams. He is involved with one important meeting after another, deals with people every minute of the day, and works long hours to keep on top of his responsibilities. He is under tremendous pressure to make sure every project gets done on time and on budget. He is also expected to keep the department overtime low, the staff morale high, and the corporate image positive. One thing is certain, John never struggles with boredom. In fact, he often wishes his job had a bit less professional stress—like Bob's.

Comparison is the enemy of contentment. It doesn't matter whether we compare our life circumstances to other people or to a master plan we've created for ourselves, the results are the same. We miss the excitement of what God is doing in our lives because we are upset over what He isn't doing. We critique His plan for our lives against the one we've drafted. When circumstances fall short we assume He is missing the mark, scarcely considering the possibility that we could be missing it instead.

HIS KINGDOM COME

Some in Jesus' day fell into the "happily ever after" trap. They expected God's plan to match their own. But when circumstances took them on a different path, they ended up surprised, disillusioned, and confused.

Life in Galilee was rather dreary for first-century men like Peter and his brother Andrew. They were ordinary fishermen, trying to scratch out a living in the midst of tough economic times. It was hard enough trying to make ends meet in the fishing trade, and Rome was making it even more difficult by demanding higher and higher taxes all the time. If after a good fishing season Peter and Andrew made a decent profit, it was eaten away by income taxes. No matter how hard they worked, it was tough to build a business beyond the mere survival stage. Needless to say, they began hating the Romans who were blocking their ability to get ahead in life.

Matthew worked for the Roman Internal Revenue Service, so he was on the other end of the tax burden. He had no trouble getting ahead financially. The Romans allowed him to enhance his income by auditing those who might have a few extra coins to spare after taxday. The more strict he was on others, the more wealthy Matthew became. In the process of becoming rich, however, he also became an outcast. Most of the Jews hated men like Matthew for betraying his own people and selling out to the Romans. They called him names like Benedict Aaron and Ezekiel Scrooge. His only friends were other outcasts of the Jewish community, tax-collectors, drunkards, and harlots. The Romans had reduced Matthew to the lowest of the low among his people, and he hated them for it.

Simon was a deeply religious man. In fact, he was part of a group so zealous over Mosaic ritual that they were nicknamed "the zealots." They loved Jewish law and custom, and were particularly upset over the Roman occupancy because it stripped Israel of its right to self-rule. It was humiliating to seek permission from a heathen governor before proceeding with religious festivals or punishing blatantly sinful acts. Simon took pride in following God's laws to the letter, and the Romans were severely cramping his style. Some of his colleagues planned to organize an insurrection with hopes of returning Israel to Jewish rule. Simon so hated the Romans that he was tempted to join them.

Happily Ever After?

In the midst of this society which was ruled by hatred and on the verge of rebellion, Jesus of Nazareth entered Galilee teaching about love and announcing the coming of a new kingdom. His timing was perfect to capture the attention of those who needed the former and wanted the latter.

Jesus was different than the many other teachers who brought a radical message to the masses—often for personal gain. He was meek, yet commanded respect. He was simple, yet deeply profound. He was comfortable around sinful people, yet lived a righteous life. He disliked the religious leaders of the day, yet taught about spiritual matters. He was unlike anything the people had ever seen before, and thousands came to learn from him. Some saw Jesus as the One who could bring meaning to their empty lives, and they left everything behind in order to follow Him. Among them were Peter, Andrew, Matthew, Simon, and eight others who became part of Jesus' inner circle of twelve.

Peter and Andrew saw Jesus as One who could make them fishers of men, and who wouldn't tax them out of business in the process. Jesus was the first person to make Matthew feel valuable without requiring that he sell out his ethics to become a somebody. Simon could hardly contain his excitement upon hearing the teachings of Jesus. Perhaps this man was the long-awaited Messiah who would finally return Israel to its rightful place of dominion in the world. Each of the twelve, for one reason or another, thought that Jesus was the answer to their hopes and prayers—the One who would overthrow Rome and establish the kingdom promised to David. Israel would once again become a great nation under the mighty and righteous rule of King Jesus—and they would live happily ever after as His comrades.

Life with Jesus started out very exciting for the twelve. It was not what they expected—it was much better. Jesus spent time with the outcasts of society, making them feel special. He made the religious establishment nervous by emphasizing love and compassion over ritual and sacrifice. He even went so far as to condemn the hypocrisy of the Pharisees, a group of pious stuff-shirts who had set themselves up as God's thought police.

Jesus performed some unbelievable miracles. He turned water into wine at a wedding celebration, made a lame man walk, gave sight to a man who had been blind since birth, and cast evil spirits out of the possessed. The word got out, and the crowds began to grow. At one point, after Jesus had been teaching all day, He decided to take a dinner break. The disciples assumed it was time to send the people away so they could grab a bite to eat. But Jesus instructed them to give the people something to eat instead. There was one big problem—they didn't even have enough food for themselves, let alone more than five thousand extra dinner guests. Still, they did as the Master told them, getting everyone seated and gathering up any food they could find. Somehow, with only two fish and a few pieces of bread, Jesus fed every person! This was the best miracle yet. It proved that this man named Jesus had every quality needed to rule Israel. Not only could He teach with power, make wine from water, heal the sick, and raise the dead, He could feed hungry people by creating food from nothing. Jesus' fame spread and the crowds continued to grow.

The disciples were getting excited about the possibilities. The best image consultant on earth couldn't have planned a better early campaign. There was no doubt in their minds that Jesus was getting ready to establish His kingdom.

Death of the Dream

Just about the time Jesus reached the peak of His popularity, He began doing some things that made the disciples a bit uneasy. Shortly after the feeding of the five thousand, for example, He started teaching about the high cost of discipleship. He said that they must be willing to reject the comforts of life and carry a cross of reproach for His name. This was a turn-off to many of Jesus' followers—so they left. He then went so far as to claim equality with God—a capital offense under Jewish law. Although the twelve were loyal and believed that Jesus had good reasons for such statements, they were concerned about what could happen to Him (and them) if word reached the envious religious leaders. The leaders wanted nothing more than to accuse Jesus of blasphemy, giving them a good reason to end this dangerous movement.

Just when things started to look grim, however, their day in the sun arrived. After more than three years of learning, watching, and waiting, the twelve entered Jerusalem with Jesus in preparation for the celebration of Passover. Huge crowds of people cheered and honored Jesus as He rode into town, proclaiming Him to be the King of Israel. The timing was perfect for Jesus to establish His kingdom. He was so popular that the people revered Him, He was so righteous that the religious leaders feared Him, and He was so powerful that nature obeyed Him. Even Rome was no match for Jesus of Nazareth.

But something went wrong. Instead of talking about potential cabinet officers for His new government, Jesus began talking about His impending death. Rather than enjoying a feast of celebration, they ate a meal which symbolized suffering. They planned to see Jesus sit on a throne, not hang on a cross. Suddenly the dream was over—their leader had been crucified as a troublemaker. One week earlier they were on top of the world, ready to overthrow Rome. Now they were the abandoned followers of a dead rebel. Frightened, confused, and disillusioned, the disciples lost all hope of living happily ever after. Jesus was dead, and so was their dream.

You know the rest of the story. Jesus rose from the dead three days later, and the disciples finally understood God's plan. Right? Wrong. They still expected Jesus to establish His kingdom and overthrow Rome. Their expectation is evident in their last question to Jesus before His return to heaven. "Lord, are you at this time going to restore the kingdom to Israel?" It was not until much later that they recognized the kingdom of God to be more than a mere earthly rule.

The disciples began following Jesus motivated by a deep hatred for Rome and the desire for greatness. But God had other plans. His "once upon a time" did not include their "happily ever after" ending. His wonderful plan for their lives was a different kind of wonderful than they could have possibly imagined. They, like we, had to reckon with the truth that God's plans for their lives may have been bigger than they expected and different than they desired.

As the disciples learned, one of the keys to contentment is accepting what God brings even when it is not what we expect. His plan is better than ours, even though we tend to view our own plan as the best possible option. Do we honestly believe that God's will for our lives is what's best for our lives? If we do, we can trust Him with our circumstances. If we don't, we had better find a different God!

Getting Personal

Have you succumbed to the myth that a place called "happily ever after" really exists? Have you been expecting some person, event, status, experience, or accomplishment to bring you into a state of permanent happiness? Have you sacrificed the certain joys of today for the uncertainties of tomorrow? Or have you accepted the possibility that God's wonderful plan for your life may not match your own wonderful plan? Why not relax by trusting Him with the reins of your life?

Chapter Four

WHEN EVERYTHING ISN'T ENOUGH

There are two tragedies in life. One is not to get your heart's desire. The other is to get it. George Bernard Shaw

Often, the things we most desire in life are least able to bring true satisfaction. We climb the ladder of success, only to discover that it is leaning against the wrong wall.

An ancient Greek fable tells of a king named Midas. Midas had more gold than anyone in the world, yet he was not satisfied. He became obsessed with the acquisition of more and more gold, and he was most happy when he entered the palace vault to count what he possessed. The only thing he loved more than gold was his young daughter, Marygold.

One day, King Midas encountered a mysterious stranger who gave him the power to turn everything he touched into gold. This made him quite happy, and he went through the palace transforming objects into gold.

Midas decided to read a book. But when he touched the edge of the cover, the book became gold. "I can't read now," he said, "but it is still much better to have a gold book than a book I can read."

When breakfast arrived, Midas reached for a piece of fresh fruit. But when he picked up the fruit, it became a lump of gold. The same happened to his glass of water. "What shall I do?" he asked. "I am hungry and thirsty, yet cannot eat or drink."

Just then Marygold came into the room with tears streaming down her cheeks. She reached out for a comforting embrace from her father, and he instinctively kissed her. To his horror, she suddenly turned into a little gold statue. King Midas screamed in anguish as he realized what he had done to the person he loved more than life itself.

Suddenly, the stranger reappeared. "Are you happy, King Midas?" he asked.

"How could I be happy?" asked the king. "I am the most miserable man alive."

"But you have the golden touch," said the stranger. "What more could you want?"

King Midas became silent in his shame.

"Please," pleaded the king, "give me back my precious Marygold and I will give up all the gold I have! I have lost all that is worth having."

"You are wiser than you were," said the stranger. After instructing the king on how to reverse his golden touch, the stranger once again vanished.

King Midas did as the stranger had instructed, and his daughter returned to life. With great joy he embraced his little girl. Never again did King Midas seek more gold, except the golden rays of the sun and little Marygold's hair.

WHAT MATTERS

One of the most difficult things to master in life is establishing and maintaining proper priorities. King Midas learned his lesson the hard way. The most important things in life were taken from him as a direct consequence of his lopsided priorities. By allowing gold to become his overriding passion, he lost all perspective on what truly matters in life.

All of us are guilty of King Midas's error. Although we may not look to gold to bring us joy, we do fall into the same pattern of lopsided priorities. We deceive ourselves into believing that we need something more than our current lot in order to attain happiness. Some may look for wealth, others status, material possessions, or countless other desires that they hope will magically bring fulfillment in life. Some people, who have learned that material goods do not bring lasting happiness, look for their ultimate satisfaction in a human relationship: a best friend, a mate, or children. And while they pursue these things, they lose sight of what really matters.

Two problems are associated with poorly placed priorities. The first is that the pursuit of future goals can rob us of present fulfillment. We are always looking around the next corner and over the next hill to find satisfaction we never fully attain. Having everything we desire is not the key to fulfillment. Rather, finding fulfillment in life is the key to enjoying what we have.

HAVING IT ALL

The search for the good life is nothing new. It is one of the oldest themes of the human experience. It has been the driving force behind mankind's best and worst accomplishments. From the horrors of slavery to the competition of capitalism, economic and political structures have been formed around the goal of making life better for some—often at the expense of others. Men and women throughout history have shared a common goal—to have it all. We want money, power, success, love, fun, and, of course, significance. Once we've acquired them all, so the theory goes, we will be satisfied. Unfortunately, few of us are able to fully test the theory because we never actually reach the goal of having it all.

TESTING THE THEORY

One man did fully test the theory and recorded his experiences for the rest of us to read. He wrote an often misunderstood little book of the Bible called Ecclesiastes. Although he failed to autograph the work, he included enough clues of his identity that most scholars believe him to be the infamous King Solomon—son of David and ruler of Israel during her glory years.

King Solomon was the wisest man of his time, and probably since. In an age when everyone wanted to know the secrets of life and the keys to success, Solomon was writing best-sellers on the topics. He ruled one of the greatest nations in the world, had obtained wealth beyond measure, and preserved peaceful prosperity for many years in a land formerly dominated by hostility and discord. Rulers from around the world came to observe his success and listen to the teachings of this expert on the art of living. Solomon was listed as "the best and brightest" and "the richest and most famous" all in one.

Having accomplished all that any man could hope, Solomon was highly qualified to address the issue of life priorities. He had it all, did it all, and knew it all. So, he set out to test whether or not the things we typically pursue in life are really worth all the effort.

Solomon began his analysis with a clear summary of his purpose. "I, the Teacher, was king over Israel in Jerusalem. I devoted myself to study and to explore by wisdom all that is done under heaven" (Ecclesiastes 1:12–13). In other words, he intended to experience everything life had to offer and evaluate those experiences with a critical eye. His aim was to complete a comprehensive analysis of life and to publish his findings for others to ponder. His dissertation found its way into the canon of Scripture, and it has since helped men and women of all ages reevaluate their priorities.

Solomon's method of evaluation was simple. He planned to experience everything firsthand. He didn't spend his time in the safety of a research library contemplating what others had said about this topic and that. Nor did he stand on the sidelines watching others play in the game of life. He jumped in with both feet to personally participate in every life experience imaginable. By the time he was finished, he was a certified expert in the science of living.

Solomon summarized his pursuits into several common categories in order to help us evaluate the merits of each. They include the pursuit of knowledge, pleasure, success, wealth, and good deeds.

Knowledge

Solomon begins his analysis with an evaluation of his personal passion, acquiring knowledge and wisdom. He had gained more than anyone else, only to discover that it doesn't bring satisfaction.

I thought to myself, "Look, I have grown and increased in wisdom more than anyone who has ruled over Jerusalem before me; I have experienced much of wisdom and knowledge." Then I applied myself to the understanding of wisdom, and also of madness and folly, but I learned that this, too, is a chasing after the wind. For with much wisdom comes much sorrow; the more knowledge, the more grief. . . . For the wise man, like the fool, will not be long remembered; in days to come both will be forgotten. Like the fool, the wise man too must die! (Ecclesiastes 1:16–18; 2:16)

It is surprising to read such an evaluation of wisdom from the man who wrote most of the book of Proverbs, in which he described knowledge as more valuable than gold and wisdom as supreme. Had Solomon become so cynical in his old age that he suddenly abandoned his earlier advice? Actually, he is not judging the value of wisdom and knowledge in and of themselves. Keep in mind, Ecclesiastes was written with a specific objective in mind—to determine whether or not the things we pursue in life bring true satisfaction. Wisdom and knowledge, as good as they may be, do not measure up. In fact, in the context of seeking fulfillment, they can become a major source of discouragement.

Do you know why ignorance is bliss? It is because we are in bondage to what we know. Sometimes it is more comfortable to remain ignorant of things we can't influence rather than become imprisoned by their disturbing images. This is the point Solomon makes after spending time in the classroom of life. It is disheartening to spend life seeking to understand the world, only to discover that it is filled with hardship, evil, and emptiness—and knowing there is nothing you can do to change it.

Knowledge does not bring fulfillment in life. Ask anyone who has spent much time in the academic world. The more you know, the more there is to learn. There is always another class to take, book to read, or paper to write. Once you've found all the answers, the questions change.

Hence, Solomon's evaluation. Understanding is far better than folly, but it falls short of bringing satisfaction in life. Although knowledge and wisdom may be the keys to success, they are not the keys to happiness.

Pleasure

Having evaluated the merits of knowledge, Solomon moves on to the pursuit of pleasure. If wisdom is not the key to fulfillment, perhaps self-gratification will do the trick. Let's read his summary.

> I thought in my heart, "Come now, I will test you with pleasure to find out what is good." But that also proved to be meaningless. "Laughter," I said, "is foolish. And what does pleasure accomplish?" I tried cheering myself with wine, and embracing folly—my mind still guiding me

with wisdom. . . . I denied myself nothing my eyes desired; I refused my heart no pleasure. (Ecclesiastes 2:1–3, 10)

If anyone had access to all forms of pleasure, it was King Solomon. He had enough wealth to buy the best food and wine, enough wives and concubines to make Hugh Hefner jealous, and enough influence to acquire the services of the best musicians, comedians, and actors in the world. He had the opportunity to experience every delight known to man, and he did. But he discovered that, despite the short-term gratification these things may bring, they do not provide the sense of deep satisfaction we seek.

God gave us the ability to enjoy certain experiences in life. He gave us tastebuds so that the necessity of eating becomes a pleasant event. He have us laughter, the most effective therapy for a discouraged heart. He gave us sex, His wonderful wedding gift to those entering a lifetime of committed love. These things are all good. But as Solomon discovered, they are not enough to bring meaning to an empty life—and often they become our downfall.

We are all capable of falling into patterns of addiction with certain vices of physical pleasure. If it is food, we live to eat rather than eat to live—slowly killing ourselves in the process. The beauty of sexual attraction turns to the filth of sexual compulsion—stealing the joy of purity from our lives. Alcohol, once merely a form of refreshment, becomes a form of bondage—destroying our lives and the lives of those we love. Entertainment changes from an activity to enjoy with friends and family to an escape from the stress of life—replacing the responsibilities of reality with the refuge of fantasy.

Pleasure is good. But it was designed with specific guidelines and limits. When we violate them in the pursuit of fulfillment, we set ourselves up for disappointment at best and devastation at worst. As Solomon saw from his own experience, "that also proved to be meaningless."

Success

One of the strongest desires we face is the passion for success. We strive to build ourselves a bigger kingdom, place more awards in the trophy case, and accumulate an index of personal achievements which will bolster our sense of identity and satisfaction—we hope. But as Solomon discovered, success can prove to be very empty.

> I undertook great projects: I built houses for myself and planted vineyards. I made gardens and parks and planted all kinds of fruit trees in them. I made reservoirs to water groves of flourishing trees. I bought male and female slaves and had other slaves who were born in my house. . . . I acquired men and women singers, and a harem as well— the delights of the heart of man. I became greater by far than anyone in Jerusalem before me. In all this my wisdom stayed with me. . . . Yet when I surveyed all that my hands had done and what I had toiled to achieve, everything was meaningless, a chasing after the wind; nothing was gained under the sun. . . . I saw that all labor and all achievement spring from man's envy of his neighbor. This too is meaningless, a chasing after the wind. (Ecclesiastes 2:4–11; 4:4)

Solomon had reached the top of the corporate ladder, climbed to the highest political office, his face appeared on the covers of both *Fortune* and *Time* magazines, and he designed and created a park rivaling the garden of Eden. Yet, after achieving all these things, he found no satisfaction.

Perhaps the most significant reason success fails to satisfy is that after each achievement, there is another hill to climb, another opportunity to pursue. There is always someone else who has done more than we have. So with each accomplishment we raise the bar of expectation, and we must jump a bit higher the next time. One success opens the opportunity for another, and another, and another. New challenges never cease, the race never ends. Though most of us would prefer winning to losing, it is difficult to know whether success is any less difficult to manage than failure. As Gilbert Brim described in his book *Ambition,*

> We all know that failure must be dealt with, but we are less likely to understand that winning brings its problems, too. When we win, the response is to increase the degree of difficulty. We set a shorter timetable for the next endeavor, raising expectations of how much we can achieve, even broadening out and adding new goals. But here's the hitch. People can become psychologically trapped by their own success as they race to keep up with the rising expectations bred by each new achievement.[1]

So what should we do? Is it best to just sit back, relax, and ignore the opportunities for achievement before us? Not at all. But we cannot allow material or business success to become our chief priority. Success will not bring satisfaction in life. As Solomon learned, we are not chasing a dream—we are chasing the wind.

Wealth

John Stuart Mill said it well. "Men do not desire to be rich, only to be richer than other men." Solomon was richer than other men, much richer: "I also owned more herds and flocks than anyone in Jerusalem before me. I amassed silver and gold for myself, and the treasure of kings and provinces" (Ecclesiastes 2:7–8).

After amassing great wealth, however, Solomon wasn't overly impressed with his balance sheet. He had learned the value of a dollar, and he discovered that it isn't very high.

> Whoever loves money never has money enough; whoever loves wealth is never satisfied with his income. This too is meaningless. As goods increase, so do those who consume them. And what benefit are they to the owner except to feast his eyes on them? . . . I have seen a grievous evil under the sun: wealth hoarded to the harm of its owner, or wealth lost through some misfortune, so that when he has a son there is nothing left for him. Naked a man comes from his mother's womb, and as he comes, so he departs. He takes nothing from his labor that he can carry in his hand. (Ecclesiastes 5:10–11, 13–15)

Solomon provides several insightful observations regarding wealth. First, if we make money a primary motivation in our lives, we will never be satisfied. The more we acquire, the more we desire. There will always be someone richer than we are, and it is precisely that person we will compare ourselves against. There will always be another sale to make, commission to earn, and deal to close. The higher our income rises, the higher our aspirations climb. The cycle never ends, and we kill ourselves trying to achieve the lifestyle we desire.

His second observation is this. Even if we were able to accumulate great wealth, what good is it? We can purchase more stuff to look at, but not much else. Possessions don't provide any added meaning in life. Increasing our net worth won't improve our self-worth. We will never accumulate more than everyone else, and they would envy us even if we could. Riches are more trouble than they are worth.

Third, Solomon notes that great wealth can have a harmful effect on its owner. On one end of the spectrum are those who allow riches to distort their priorities to the point that they neglect the more important aspects of life—much like King Midas. On the other end are those who allow the intoxication of wealth to overtake sound judgment. Finally possessing enough money to join the lifestyles of the rich and famous, they end up living in self-indulgent misery. Either way, as Solomon warns, the wealth they obtain leads down a path of warped priorities and personal harm.

Finally, even if you are able to avoid the pitfalls of fortune, there is still the very real possibility that you could lose everything. Wealth is fleeting. A single tragedy, robbery, or economic collapse could empty your bank account in no time at all. Happiness that depends upon riches is at best a short-term satisfaction, and at worst a veiled grief.

Good Deeds

If knowledge, pleasure, success, and wealth fail to provide fulfillment in this life, perhaps the answer lies in dedicating ourselves to a life of good deeds. Maybe by championing the cause of the less fortunate we will go to our deaths knowing our lives were worth something. Maybe if we avoid evil and promote virtue, we will be rewarded with a deep sense of satisfaction in having lived a righteous life. Maybe by promoting important causes we will find personal significance and joy. But then again, maybe not.

> So I reflected on all this and concluded that the righteous and the wise and what they do are in God's hands, but no man knows whether love or hate awaits him. All share a common destiny—the righteous and the wicked, the good and the bad, the clean and the unclean, those who offer sacrifices and those who do not. . . . This is the evil in everything that happens under the sun: The same destiny overtakes all. (Ecclesiastes 9:1–3)

We can spend our lives doing noble deeds, promoting good causes, and helping the less fortunate, but we still end up facing the same earthly destiny as the stingy reprobate. If we look at earth only, doing good deeds brings only temporary satisfaction. After a few obligatory remarks from friends and family, we will be lowered into the ground—to be forgotten shortly thereafter. Some will leave a more positive legacy than others, but the fact that they must leave it is the same for all.

In light of our mortality and God's ultimate control over all things, any contribution we can make to the world is relatively insignificant. Don't get me wrong, it is far better to spend life serving others than serving ourselves. But it is often difficult to separate the two. We often reach out to others in order to ease a guilty conscience or to convince ourselves that we are good. We need to feel needed, and we want to feel noble. But, as Solomon discovered, we must eventually reckon with the reality that life rewards the good and the bad with the same end—death. We know from other passages in Scripture that believers in Christ have a different ultimate future than unbelievers do, but nevertheless, doing good deeds for their own sake has a limited sense of fulfillment.

Another reason that good deeds are unable to provide the sense of contentment we seek is that there is always more to do. There are always more needy people than we can help, always more causes to support than money to give, and always more right things to do than time to do them. Just as those who are trying to gain riches can never acquire enough money, we can never do enough good things. Good deeds should be seen as admirable, but not as the key to personal fulfillment.

The Verdict

Without going into every aspect of Solomon's summary, it should be noted that the balance of Ecclesiastes paints a painfully honest portrait of human experience. Take the time to read this entire book, and you will find that he thoroughly tested the theory of more is better, ending his report with an abrupt but profound conclusion: "Now all has been heard; here is the conclusion of the matter: Fear God and keep his commandments, for this is the whole duty of man" (Ecclesiastes 12:13).

Contentment and satisfaction do not come from having it all. They don't even come from doing the right things. They come, according to Solomon, from a proper perspective of who God is. Throughout the book of Ecclesiastes, Solomon lived as a man seeking satisfaction independent of God. He was the master of his own destiny and the center of his universe. He submitted to no rules or limitations and denied himself no pleasure or possession. He was, so to speak, his own god. As a result, none of the things he accomplished, acquired, or enjoyed brought any lasting satisfaction. He had everything, did everything, and knew everything—only to discover just how empty such an existence can be.

Solomon made the same mistake as King Midas. Both allowed their desires to become their god. The appetite for more caused them to lose perspective on what really matters in life. The pursuit of knowledge, pleasure, success, wealth or good deeds is not wrong. In fact, properly placed, such pursuits can bring a great deal of enjoyment and satisfaction in life. The minute they become our primary focus, however, they push us further away from the contentment we hope they will provide.

Solomon's experiences reveal two important principles. First, if our priorities are not properly placed, then everything will not be enough. We typically view contentment as a prize at the end of our race for more. But contentment is a journey, not a destination. Until we are able to embrace this reality, we will never arrive. Second, understanding and trusting God's sovereign control will keep our priorities properly placed. We will look closer at this principle later as we examine the power of perspective.

It is not until our priorities and perspective are properly aligned with what really matters in life that we can find a place called enough.

THE STATE OF ENOUGH

Webster defines the word "enough" in this way: *As much or as many as necessary, desirable, or tolerable; sufficient.* Based upon this definition, we can assume that once we attain a certain level of stuff, status, or money, we reach the state of enough.

I'm afraid I have some bad news. All the money in the world, the most wonderful man or woman in the world, or the most successful career in the world can never get you to the state of enough. You can accomplish every goal, fulfill every fantasy, and surpass your wildest dreams, and still be miles away from the state of enough. I also have some good news. You can have none of these things and be very close to it. In fact, you may have a better chance at reaching the state of enough than those who have it all.

What is the state of enough? First, the state of enough is the place in life where you stop hoping that someday will bring you happiness—and you begin finding happiness today. It is the place where joy no longer depends upon circumstances but on satisfaction with what God has given you.

Second, the state of enough is the place where you take personal responsibility for what you can change, and relinquish responsibility for what you can't. There is a vast difference between finding contentment in the midst of circumstances you can't control and passively accepting those you can. Understanding this difference is the key to finding the balance between accepting and improving your lot in life. In the state of enough, you are content with what you are unable to change about your life, even if it is not what you would choose.

Finally, the state of enough is a place of rest. It is allowing yourself the freedom to stop the endless pursuit of more and better, and to rest from the heavy burden of dissatisfaction. It is the place in life where you can look at what you have, who you are, and what you do, and finally smile in approval.

The state of enough is, quite simply, the place of contentment. And once you've reached it, you will never want to go back.

Getting Personal

Have you bought into the theory which says that acquiring enough stuff, status, and money will bring fulfillment? Have you discovered that having everything is not enough? Are you ready to lighten your load? If so, come with me as we examine the art of contentment.

NOTE

1. Gilbert Brim, *Ambition: How to Manage Success and Failure Throughout Our Lives* (New York: Basic, 1992), 30–32.

Part Two

. . . .

THE PRACTICE
OF CONTENTMENT

Chapter Five

THE
LOST ART

Contentment is natural wealth, luxury is artificial poverty.
Socrates

I have come to realize that contentment is not a status to reach, but rather a discipline to learn. It is not unlike the work of an artist who invests many hours of painstaking effort to create his masterpiece. Great works of art are not thrown together quickly by someone in a hurry to achieve success. They are given the time and attention necessary to earn a place on the museum wall.

Michelangelo spent several years lying flat on his back, giving careful attention to thousands of tedious details in order to create the glorious ceiling of the Sistine Chapel. It was a labor of love, the end result being one of the most magnificent accomplishments in the history of art. But it was a labor. Discipline was the key ingredient. Had Michelangelo allowed impatience or boredom to overtake his spirit, the Sistine Chapel ceiling would have probably ended up an off-white semi-gloss.

Perhaps you know some people who are walking masterpieces of content living. They somehow maintain a sense of fulfillment regardless of circumstance. When things go well, they are grateful. When life falls apart, they hold together. They are able to accept good and bad without losing their joy or sacrificing their priorities.

My goal

They are a work of art to behold, and an example to model. That doesn't mean that strong Christians don't struggle during hard times. In fact, hard times prove how weak even the strongest of us are; we can survive only by leaning on God. But through the difficulties faith is tested and grows stronger.

A WOMAN OF SIMPLICITY

My great-grandmother Horan lived one mile from our home in the suburbs of Detroit. Although I didn't realize it at the time, I was quite blessed to have spent much of my childhood in her company. She was part of a vanishing breed that had learned to master contentment, and my life was enriched through her example.

Great-grandmother began her life in a small Indiana town during the late 1890s. She was the oldest of ten children—a very large family by our standards, but common in her day. Turn-of-the-century farm life required a tremendous amount of work, so children were considered a blessing, not a burden. Everyone, kids included, knew how to pitch in. Hard work was a way of life for great-grandmother and her nine siblings. As the oldest, things became particularly tough for her after her mother died—making it necessary that she tend to the other children and oversee most household chores. She had to grow up quickly in an age when childhood was already brief. After years serving as substitute mother for her siblings, she married and started a family of her own.

If her childhood was difficult, Grandma's early adult life was worse. She and her husband endured the hardships of the Great Depression, scratching out a living for their three children in an era when mere survival was success. Food and housing were not taken for granted but considered blessings. Instead of pursuing what they lacked, they learned to enjoy what they had. My great-grandmother somehow found the secret of contentment despite little material wealth, or maybe because of it. I never once heard her complain or reflect negatively upon the hardships she had endured. She maintained a spirit of gratitude and satisfaction even though hers had been a difficult life.

Life started simple for my grandma, and she was happy to keep it that way. Her childhood was spent in a world without automobiles, fast-food restaurants, prime-time television, or nine-to-five schedules. She never found much use for any of these things even in her later years. Surrounded by all the gadgets and conveniences of modern life, she maintained a simple existence. She rarely left home, with the exception of an annual trip to her family reunion in Indiana. She spent most of her time tending a small garden in the yard or sitting in front of an old radio listening to her favorite preachers. Her primary diet consisted of fresh vegetables from the garden, fried eggs at breakfast, and fried chicken at dinner. (Apparently fried foods did not become a health hazard until our generation—she lived to be over ninety.) The color television set in her sitting room accumulated more dust than viewing time. Her house, built by her late husband, was small and plain. She had no dishwashing machine, garbage disposal, or microwave.

I'll tell you why. My great-grandmother had found the natural wealth of contentment, so she had no need for luxury. Her life was just fine as it was, thank you. She gave little thought to fancier things, better circumstances, or a higher income. Instead, she fostered a spirit of gratitude for the simple pleasures of a simple life. My grandmother had reached the place of enough. As a result, she was a masterpiece of contentment and a model of how to find fulfillment apart from having it all.

WHAT IS CONTENTMENT?

Before we can foster contentment in our lives, we must understand what it is. Webster says that it is having or showing no desire for something more or different. Someone else said that contentment is not the fulfillment of what you want, but the realization of how much you already have. Both are pretty good definitions. But we need more. Fortunately, a man during the early days of the church had become quite an expert on the topic, and he provided some key insights for our benefit.

I Have Learned . . .

The apostle Paul knew precisely what it takes to master contentment, and he understood the benefits of doing so. He confronted the disappointment of unmet expectations as well as the enticement of endless opportunity. But he did not allow either to distort his priorities or steal his joy. Paul described his personal journey toward contented living in a letter to the church at Philippi.

Paul wrote his letter to the Philippians while under Roman house arrest, awaiting his trial and possible execution. After discovering that Paul had been imprisoned, the Christians at Philippi took up a collection and delivered it to him. Grateful for their concern and tangible expression of love, Paul sent a thank-you note. He used the occasion to include some helpful thoughts about how to maintain a sense of joy despite unpleasant circumstances—a subject on which Paul had become quite an expert. Years earlier it was in their very city that Paul was arrested, beaten, and thrown in jail for preaching the gospel. He knew firsthand what it was like to expect the best, only to experience the worst. Yet he was able to say honestly that he had found the secret to contentment:

> I have learned to be content whatever the circumstances. I know what it is to be in need, and I know what it is to have plenty. I have learned the secret of being content in any and every situation, whether well fed or hungry, whether living in plenty or in want. I can do everything through him who gives me strength. (Philippians 4:11–13)

Considering that Paul was under Roman guard and in the midst of some very unpleasant circumstances at the time he wrote this, he was not uttering empty platitudes, but telling the honest condition of his heart. Let's examine several elements of Paul's confession which help us better understand the what and how of true contentment.

(1) First, contentment is a learned discipline. Paul did not say that he discovered, stumbled across, or manufactured contentment in his life. He said that he had *learned* the secret of being content in any situation. If it can be learned, it is within reach for all of us. Paul did not have a naturally contented personality, making it easier for him than for others. Just ask John Mark, Barnabas, and others who encountered his stubborn resolve. Nor did he reach some mystical spiritual status which gave him an advantage over the rest of us. He learned it through the school of hard knocks. And so must we.

(2) Second, contentment is found apart from external factors. Paul did not depend upon other people or circumstances for his satisfaction. The word translated "content" in this passage suggests the con-

cept of sufficiency. In other words, we can maintain a sense of contentment apart from factors external to ourselves. It is an internal attitude of discipline that we develop, not a position that we reach. Paul had experienced poverty and wealth, eating well and going hungry, the praise of men and the stones of an angry mob. He endured both good and bad, maintaining a deep sense of satisfaction throughout. Based upon Paul's example, we can foster contentment in life regardless of our specific circumstances. But we must learn to stop relying upon other people, material wealth, status, or any other external factor to bring us the contentment we seek.

3 Third, contentment is not the same as apathy. Notice that Paul says he has learned to be content *in* every situation—not *with* every situation. There is a vast difference between being satisfied despite circumstances and becoming passively indifferent to them. It is foolish to deny the negative aspects of life or artificially manufacture a false sense of satisfaction with them. True contentment is the ability to honestly face the bad without allowing it to rob us of our joy. It is possible to desire a change in circumstances while maintaining a deep sense of peace and contentment in the midst of them. We can't depend upon an ideal marriage for fulfillment. But it is right to seek counseling when marital problems arise. Don't expect your job to make you rich. But if your salary isn't enough to meet your family needs, find a better one. Don't confuse contentment with complacency. Seek to improve your circumstances, but at the same time don't let them undermine your joy.

4 Fourth, contentment helps us to endure hardship. Paul said that he could do all things through Jesus, the One who gave him strength. Another way of putting it would be, 'I can cope with anything, good or bad, as long as I am trusting in the Lord.' Why? Because Paul had traded self-sufficiency for Christ's sufficiency. His joy came from relationship with an unchanging God, not reaction to continually changing circumstances. As Paul had learned, life is rarely easy, and often it is difficult. Until we are willing to adjust to this reality, difficulty will throw us off balance, rob us of our joy, and drive us to bitterness. Paul was able to cope with anything life threw his way—not because he was such a great man, but because he depended upon a great God.

The Love of Money

Paul had more to say about contentment in a letter he wrote to his young apprentice, Timothy. After a caution about those who build a great ministry for the sake of financial gain, he went on to outline a better perspective for Timothy and for us. "But godliness with contentment is great gain. For we brought nothing into the world, and we can take nothing out of it. But if we have food and clothing, we will be content with that. People who want to get rich fall into temptation and a trap and into many foolish and harmful desires that plunge men into ruin and destruction. For the love of money is a root of all kinds of evil. Some people, eager for money, have wandered from the faith and pierced themselves with many griefs." (1 Timothy 6:6–10)

How do we avoid the pitfalls of the money trap? With godly contentment. How do we keep the desire for more from warping our priorities? With godly contentment. How do we avoid piercing ourselves with many griefs? With godly contentment. In short, the love of money (things) drives us into misery, whereas the love of God drives us to contentment. Unfortunately, that principle is simple to understand, but hard to adopt. Our natural tendency is to want more, more, more. It is like the world is holding out a big chocolate-chip cookie for the taking, and the Lord tells us to be content with the celery stick we already have. Sure, we know celery is better for us in the long run. But that cookie sure looks more tasty! The desire for something better is often at the root of self-destruction. As Paul warned Timothy, those who desire bigger and better "fall into temptation and a trap and into many foolish and harmful desires that plunge men into ruin and destruction." But when we develop and maintain a sense of godly contentment, we avoid many of the pitfalls of life.

The story is told of a man and his wife who had the good fortune to possess a goose that laid one golden egg every day. They were lucky to have such a steady means toward achieving wealth, but they soon began to think that they were not getting rich quickly enough. So, thinking that the bird must be made of gold on the inside, they decided to kill it in order to get at the whole store of gold at once. But when they cut it open they discovered that it was just like

92

any other goose. Thus, they neither got rich quickly, as they had hoped, nor enjoyed any longer the daily addition to their wealth.[1]

This is Paul's caution to Timothy, as well as the rest of us. In the process of trying to get rich we make ourselves poor because we lose the ability to enjoy what we have, With contentment, enough is everything. Without contentment, everything is not enough, and that is an unhappy way to live.

The Practice of Contentment

What then is true contentment? First, it is a learned discipline—any of us can achieve it regardless of status. Second, it does not depend on external circumstances, but can be fostered in the midst of any situation. Consequently, nothing has to transpire before we can pursue content living. Third, contentment is not the same as apathy. Whether or not you are a passive person is irrelevant. Like Paul, we can have aggressive personalities and motivations, yet still learn contentment. In short, contentment is an active discipline, which we learn apart from external factors such as circumstances, status, or possessions. It fosters an abiding sense of satisfaction whether or not our expectations are fulfilled. Sounds simple, right? Well, maybe not.

Note that our ability to master contentment is heavily dependent upon a strong spiritual commitment. We cannot separate how we respond to the circumstances of life from how we relate to the Author of life. Theologian J. I. Packer has said, "The comprehensiveness of our contentment is another measure whereby we may judge whether we really know God." In other words, true contentment depends upon a proper perception of and relationship with God.

Sadly, we tend to artificially separate religious devotion from the practical realities of daily life. We want God as a hobby. It is fine to believe, but not to the point that we let our faith influence the important matters of life. And yet, we can only maintain a healthy perspective on the expectations and disappointments of life when we have a solid spiritual foundation. Even though the tenets of our faith won't change our circumstances, they can help us see them from a better perspective—something we desperately need. As we will learn from the words of Jesus, until our spiritual priorities are properly aligned, it is impossible to experience the quiet rest of contentment.

All These Things

It would be interesting, and depressing, to track just how much time and energy we spend fretting over things. We worry about getting what we lack, keeping what we have, and losing what we don't really need. I often wonder what God must think of such silly concerns. Well, in the midst of His famous Sermon on the Mount, Jesus spent a few minutes talking about this very issue. After some straight talk on proper priorities, He made several powerful statements that give us a heavenly perspective on all these things: "Do not worry about your life, what you will eat or drink; or about your body, what you will wear. Is not life more important than food, and the body more important than clothes? Look at the birds of the air; they do not sow or reap or store away in barns, and yet your heavenly Father feeds them. Are you not much more valuable than they? Who of you by worrying can add a single hour to his life?" (Matthew 6:25–27).

If all the research about stress is correct, worrying will not add an hour to life—it will take one away. Many a heart attack has been caused by anxiety over buying a bigger house, driving a better car, and climbing the corporate ladder. There is too much to accomplish to sit back and enjoy life. Meanwhile, a bird perches itself on a branch outside our window and sings a simple song. From God's perspective, the bird has the right idea.

Christ goes on to address another topic that people often worry about: "And why do you worry about clothes? See how the lilies of the field grow. They do not labor or spin. Yet I tell you that not even Solomon in all his splendor was dressed like one of these. If that is how God clothes the grass of the field, which is here today and tomorrow is thrown into the fire, will he not much more clothe you, O you of little faith?" (Matthew 6:28–30).

Is Jesus suggesting that we quit our jobs, abandon our responsibilities, and join a nudist colony? Hardly. He is simply pointing out the futility of worry in light of God's ability to meet our needs. He is also touching upon something very important to each of us—our wardrobe. What we wear says a lot about our priorities. As does what we drive, where we live, and how we spend our money. In short, we invest too much energy in things that are not evil, but which can easily distract us from what truly matters. In fact, Jesus equates such concerns with the life of a pagan. "So do not worry, saying, 'What shall we eat?' or 'What shall we drink?' or 'What shall we wear?' For the pagans run after all these things, and your heavenly Father knows that you need them" (Matthew 6:31–32).

You see, those who have no relationship with God are limited to the shallow satisfaction which comes from things. With no lasting basis for joy, they are left to seek fulfillment from temporal pleasures and material possessions. The believer, on the other hand, has access to a far greater source of meaning in life. That is why Jesus goes on to say, "But seek first his kingdom and his righteousness, and all these things will be given to you as well" (Matthew 6:33).

Some have misinterpreted Jesus' words at this point as a promise of perpetual wealth and prosperity for all believers. Wrong! The context is one of meeting our basic needs, not satisfying our every desire. Jesus' point is that it is foolish to worry about "all these things" when there is a greater source of joy in life. He may very well give us the things we want. More importantly, He can help us view them for what they are—just things.

Unfortunately, in our culture of affluence it is difficult to maintain such a healthy perspective. According to Richard Foster, the reason is that we have lost what he calls the freedom of simplicity.

> Contemporary culture is plagued by the passion to possess. The unreasoned boast abounds that the good life is found in accumulation, that "more is better." Indeed, we often accept this notion without question, with the result that the lust for affluence in contemporary society has become psychotic: it has completely lost touch with reality. Furthermore, the pace of the modern world accentuates our sense of being fractured and fragmented. We feel strained, hurried, breathless. The complexity of rushing to achieve and accumulate more and more frequently threatens to overwhelm us; it seems there is no escape from the rat race.[2]

He's right. We stop wanting what we have in the process of pursuing what we want. Somewhere along the way we lose sight of what is truly important. And before long we begin making unhealthy choices and breeding unnecessary stress in our lives.

An incredible freedom comes when we learn to want what we have. When we let them, the simple pleasures of life can replace the need for bigger and better. They allow us to feel rich without having it all. Unfortunately, few of us have discovered the secret to obtaining such quiet peace in our lives. The drive for more and better keeps us moving forward, but never brings us the satisfaction we seek. We continue to make ourselves poor with the quest for more and to make ourselves miserable due to ill-placed priorities. But it doesn't have to be that way. If contentment is a discipline rather than a status, it is available to all.

MASTERING CONTENTMENT

Now that we have a better handle on the definition of contentment, we are left with a lingering question—How do we get it? It does us little good to understand the what if we don't know the how. We have defined the goal, but not the road to getting there. How do we move beyond the desire to master the art and start creating our own masterpiece? The later chapters of this book will attempt to answer this question.

Mastering any skill requires understanding the fundamentals. Before we can create a master painting, we must learn to use a paint brush. Before competing in a PGA tournament, we must learn to hold a golf club. Before writing the great American novel, we must learn the alphabet. In every area of life there are basic disciplines which must be understood and practiced before we can achieve success. The same is true with contentment. None of us wakes up one morning and suddenly enters a state of perpetual satisfaction. Reaching and maintaining contentment is a never-ending struggle. There are no magic words or simple formulas. It is a daily choice undergirded by an ongoing commitment. Like anything worthwhile, it requires persistence. But it is more than worth the effort.

Before we can begin, it is important to understand that contentment is not a direct target, but an indirect benefit. We will be highlighting several attitudes and habits which indirectly foster contentment in our lives. As we will discover, we cannot eliminate the negative impact of unmet expectations. We can, however, overshadow them with a deep sense of fulfillment.

In later chapters we will be thoroughly examining the factors which breed contentment. However, I will briefly mention each at this point in order to focus our attention in the right direction.

THE FACTORS WHICH BREED CONTENTMENT:

Identity: Low self-worth severely undermines contentment. If our identity depends on status, possessions, or relationships, we will never fully find the sense of fulfillment we seek.

Perspective: How we see the circumstances of life will drive how we respond to them. So it is important to develop a perspective which allows us to rest in God's ultimate control over the particular aspects of living.

Comparison: Comparing our situation to others will undermine contentment faster than anything. We need to recognize the impact of the comparison game in order to avoid its curse in our lives.

Gratitude: When we develop an ongoing habit of gratitude, we foster a sense of contentment even when our expectations are unfulfilled. A grateful heart is never poor.

These four form the fundamentals of our discipline. We must understand and properly align each before we can master contentment. Every one of them has the potential of undermining or fostering contentment. When we learn to make them work for us rather than against us, their collective impact can revolutionize our lives.

One final thought before we roll up our sleeves and dig into the "how to" of this subject: The pursuit of contentment is a never-ending process. Once mastered, the discipline must be maintained. Even concert pianists must practice or they will regress into mediocre musicians. The greatest Olympic athletes of all time will become couch potatoes if they neglect the discipline of exercise. The same is true with the art of contentment. Once mastered, it must be continually maintained. It is a discipline, not a status. But it is more than worth the effort.

Getting Personal

Have you considered contentment a status to reach or an attitude to cultivate? Have you learned the discipline of finding contentment apart from external circumstances? Can you maintain a sense of satisfaction in the midst of any situation? If you want to cultivate attitudes and habits in your life which will foster rather than undermine contentment, follow me as we move forward on our quest.

NOTES

1. Aesop's fable as retold by William J. Bennett, *The Book of Virtues* (New York: Simon & Schuster, 1993), 47.

2. Richard J. Foster, *Freedom of Simplicity* (San Francisco: Harper Collins, 1981), 3.

Chapter Six

THE IMPACT OF IDENTITY

A lot of people don't realize they have an identity crisis until they try to cash a check in a strange town.
Bill Vaughn

Sarah walked into the room where I was waiting to interview her for a job. It was evident immediately that she didn't like herself, that she felt unworthy. Her appearance and demeanor spoke volumes. As we talked, my initial impressions were confirmed. Sarah was in her early forties, a bit overweight, never married, and never happy. She had moved from one unfulfilling job to another, and now she wanted to work with a Christian ministry, hoping to find the satisfaction she craved. She had a strong set of professional skills and a very sharp wit—apparently developed as a coping mechanism. She poked fun at herself as if she wanted to highlight her flaws before another person had time to notice them. Her forced grin failed to hide what she truly felt—"Please don't reject me." I gave Sarah the job, and she has become a successful employee. But she still doesn't like herself, and she still craves satisfaction.

Paul can't understand why everything seems to go wrong in his life. He works hard, but he never gets promoted. He is nice to others, but he has few friends. He attends church and sings about "showers of blessings," but they never fall in his own life. If Paul buys a car, it is sure to be a lemon. If he is attracted to a woman, she will only want to be friends. If he does anything outstanding at work, someone else will get the credit. In short, nothing goes right for Paul—he is a perpetual victim. At least that's what Paul says. If you have a conversation with him, plan on hearing about another mishap or disappointment. He is constantly discouraged and sees failure as an inevitable part of his generally worthless existence. Oh, and don't bother trying to cheer him up. Paul is convinced that gloom and calamity are his lot in life.

When Tammy walks your direction, you can kiss your plans for the hour good-bye. She will talk, and talk, and talk some more. Of course, the entire conversation will center on Tammy—her latest accomplishment, or her latest purchase, or her latest trauma. And if you happen to be someone she considers important, watch out! She will dominate your time and monopolize your attention. Hanging out with important people gives her something to talk about when she is with others. Tammy can drive you crazy without even trying. But those who look past the front and listen through the chatter will discover more: Tammy is desperately lonely. She longs for someone to want her, to accept her, to love her. She talks about herself because she lacks the confidence to talk about anything else. Unfortunately, in her effort to gain the acceptance of others, she is driving them farther away. She has become her own worst enemy.

Bill drives an expensive sports car. He is very handsome, has a lovely wife, lives in the elite part of town, and wears the latest fashions. Bill owns his own business and makes a lot of money. He appears to have it all together. But Bill is not happy. His possessions, appearance, and image effectively mask a carefully-kept secret—Bill is searching for something that will give him joy. He has worked hard to build a perfect world for himself, only to discover that it can't fill the void deep within his heart. So his pursuit continues. Bill will buy an even more expensive car. He will make even more money. He will move into an even nicer home. And he will remain unhappy.

What do Sarah, Paul, Tammy, and Bill all have in common? In two words—poor identity. The symptoms of their struggle are different, but the root issue is the same. How we perceive ourselves has a direct influence upon our level of satisfaction in life. Those who develop a healthy sense of identity will find the road to contentment much easier than those who don't. No matter how much we possess

THE IMPACT OF IDENTITY

or what status we reach, how we see ourselves is a critical element to finding any lasting sense of contentment.

Sarah sees herself as a worthless, unattractive woman who fails to measure up in a society that values a perfect figure and cover-girl smile. So she laughs to cover her tears.

Paul sees himself as a victim to the unfairness of life. So he moans and groans in response to his misery.

Tammy sees herself as all alone in the world, unaccepted by those around her. So she throws herself at others, hoping they will notice her and think she is special.

Bill sees himself as king of the mountain. He deserves the best things in life, and he intends to have them all. So he fills his castle with a bunch of neat stuff, but he is unable to fill the void in his heart.

All of us, to one degree or another, struggle with our sense of identity. We have been programmed since childhood to measure our worth against the things that this world considers important. Those who don't measure up spend life feeling unworthy. Even those who do measure up quickly discover it doesn't satisfy—that they've been striving for the wrong things.

As long as our sense of identity depends on a good job, an attractive body, a large house, a fancy car, or any other temporal thing, we will never feel satisfied. True contentment is first and foremost a spiritual issue.

So what's the answer? How do we break the cycle of dissatisfaction and emptiness? We must first understand the impact of identity. We must clearly and accurately define who we are, what we need, and what it takes to get it.

THE SEARCH

Whenever I go to a mall I typically try to avoid casually strolling from one retail outlet to another, because if I wander I end up buying more than I intended. My goal is to walk directly to the store I need, get in and get out as quickly as possible—do not pass go, do not spend two hundred dollars. (Unless, of course, I happen across a bookstore.)

Not long ago I went to a shopping mall in search of a particular store. I wanted to purchase a specific item, and I knew which store carried it. After walking into the mall's side entrance, I was confronted with row after row of stores—big stores, small stores, clothing stores, shoestores, bookstores, art stores, exercise-equipment stores, novelty stores, game stores, even a junk-food store or two. I had a problem. Since I had only been in the mall once or twice before, I did not know the layout or which direction would lead me to the store I needed. So I did what any bewildered shopper would do—I began walking down the first row. Two hours later, I had spent all my money and forgotten what it was I needed.

If I had been smart, I would have gone directly to the mall layout map and looked for those wonderful words, "You are here." I then could have traced my path from where I was to where I needed to be. That simple step could have saved me wasted time and a busted budget.

The same is true when it comes to personal identity. When we fail to understand and develop a healthy sense of identity, it is like skipping the "you are here" sign at the mall. We lose sight of who we are and what it is that we truly need. The void is quickly filled by one or more of the things that promise meaning in life. "More stuff available here!" shouts one marquee. "Beauty and fame this way!" promises another. "Pamper yourself—you deserve it" says a third. "Discipline yourself—you need it" declares a fourth. We waste a lot of time and energy trying it all, and we forget what it was we needed along the way.

In order to find that which will truly satisfy, we must locate the "you are here" dot on the proverbial map of life. We need something to show us where we stand in the greater scheme of things. Are we in the center of the map or in a remote location? Do we have a long way to go before reaching our destination, or is it just around the corner? Is our actual location anywhere near the place we think we've been standing?

More often than not, we skip the "you are here" process and jump right into the endless pursuit of fulfillment. We walk up and down the corridors of life trying to find something that will satisfy. We try possessions, but they don't do it. We try popularity, but find it fleeting. We try pleasure, but the void remains. As many have discovered, we will come up empty-handed unless we are willing to pause long enough to identify what it is we are looking for and where we must go to get it.

You see, by intentionally defining who we are and what we need, we are better equipped to actively pursue that which will satisfy. There is a void inside, we all know that. But we also need to know its shape so that we can properly fill it. Where we have no clear game plan, the void will be filled by whatever the world throws our way. We end up with plenty of "stuff" in our lives, but no lasting satisfaction. Taking time out to find the "you are here" marker on the map will place us on the right path.

WHICH MAP?

In a shopping mall, there is one reference map. In real life, there are countless versions of the map, all claiming to accurately represent the world and our place in it. These maps are known as worldviews. Each worldview offers its own version of who we are, how the world operates, and what will bring us happiness. Let's briefly touch upon some of the predominant worldviews and how they define our relationship to God and our personal identity.

"There Is No God"

There are very few true atheists. Most rational individuals discovered a long time ago that a godless worldview is bankrupt and ill-reasoned. Yet, many still live as if God does not exist—as if we are on our own in the endless search for purpose in life. "If God does exist," so the theory goes, "He certainly doesn't care about the petty details of our lives."

What does the "you are here" marker of this worldview suggest? It says that you and I are little more than animals caught in the struggle to survive. Life has no meaning beyond personal gratification, and happiness is found through indulgence. In short, this perspective offers no true contentment because we can only fill the emptiness on a temporary basis—moving from one pleasure to the next in the endless pursuit of satisfaction. The void remains.

"You Are God"

Another prominent worldview has been labeled "New Age"— but it is actually not new at all. Pantheism, upon which the New Age Movement is built, has been around for thousands of years. Rather than "there is no God," this perspective says "you are God." Everything is God and God is everything. Rather than a personal being with whom we can relate, God is an impersonal force of which we are a part. What is important is that we release our individuality and become part of the greater whole. Fulfillment comes from within because we are the true source of wisdom and power. We do not depend on anything outside ourselves for satisfaction or deliverance. If we go within ourselves and find that which we've lost, we can discover our own godhood in the process.

What does this "you are here" marker tell us? It says we should abandon personal identity and the search for meaning in life and replace it with the realization of our own godhood. We can go within to find truth. We can go within to find meaning. We can go within to find ultimate fulfillment. We don't need to find God; we are God! Sadly, many spend their entire lives looking within for the god of self when what they really need is relationship with the God of heaven. The void remains.

"God Is Gonna Getcha"

Even those worldviews built upon the understanding of God as an all-powerful creator can portray Him differently. The "God is gonna getcha" view, for example, says that God is a cold-hearted, angry fellow. He spends His time peering down upon a disobedient world, hoping to catch someone doing wrong so that He can zap him with one of His favorite punishments—like sickness, poverty, death, or the ultimate zap—eternal damnation. He demands absolute obedience and places unreasonable demands upon His servants. So millions dutifully participate in regimented religious ritual and avoid pleasurable activities in order to avoid His wrath.

This worldview tells us to watch our step. It says that God is eagerly anticipating the day we fail so that He can give us what we deserve. It says that we should live in fear and restrict our joy. It says that we had better be good or else! In short, it tells us we are unloved and unworthy. The void remains.

"God—at Your Service"

On the other extreme are those who view God as little more than a powerful bellhop or a giant genie in a bottle. His role is to

THE IMPACT OF IDENTITY

jump at every faith-filled wish to make our every dream come true. "If God truly loves His children," so they say, "He will give them what they want." When God fails to pull through, we cram Him back in the bottle and reject His false promises. (Promises, by the way, that He never made.)

What does this map tell us about who we are and what we need? It says that God owes us something—namely, the good life. It says that we are the center of the universe—God's ultimate focus. If poor little Billy is hurting, God is obligated to run to his aid. If Sally is sad, of course God will give her the things that she thinks will make her happy. We deserve what we want because we are God's spoiled kids. And if He doesn't give them to us, we will just take our faith and go home! The void remains.

None of these worldviews, or life maps, leads us to where we want to go. They present themselves as accurate representations of the world and our place in it, but they give us faulty directions. They may contain elements of truth, but none of them hits the mark. Fortunately, I have good news. God has given us an accurate map to follow. Within the pages of the Bible we will find everything we need to establish an identity based upon reality. It clearly points out our place in the world and where we need to go to find the satisfaction we seek. Why wander aimlessly through the mall of life when we can locate the "you are here" marker as described by the Master designer Himself?

YOU ARE HERE

It is impossible to find contentment apart from a healthy sense of identity. It is critical that we develop an accurate perception of who we are. Let's look at several key scriptural truths that will help us understand ourselves from God's perspective a little better. Most importantly, we are . . .

Made in God's Image

It's a familiar story. God created the world in six days, leaving His final creative masterpiece for last—mankind. Adam and Eve were made in God's own image. Unlike any other creature, they were given the ability to reason, invent, build, organize, and develop. Most significant, however, was their will. Man was uniquely endowed with the ability to choose right or wrong, good or bad, relationship with or rejection of God. Adam and Eve were free to choose to love God, which is the basis of real relationship. They were not forced, but invited. It was wonderful at first. They walked with the Lord in Paradise, living in perfect harmony with their world and their Creator. Everything was ideal, until they sinned and ended up . . .

Separated from God

Prompted by temptation, man chose to reject God's protective authority. Enticed by the possibility of becoming his own master, Adam abandoned relationship with his Creator. That choice summarizes the tragedy of the human experience. Though created with a capacity for relationship with God, and instilled with a need for relationship with God, we reject Him. Hence, the void within. As C. S. Lewis put it:

> God designed the human machine to run on Himself. He Himself is the fuel our spirits were designed to burn, or the food our spirits were designed to feed on. There is no other. That is why it is just no good asking God to make us happy in our own way without bothering about religion. God cannot give us a happiness and peace apart from Himself, because it is not there. There is no such thing.[1]

The moment we reject His plan is the moment we abandon true, lasting joy. That is what Adam did in the Garden, and what the rest of us have done as well. Life is no longer as it should be because we are . . .

Fallen

When man pulled himself out from under God's authority, he also rejected the opportunity to live life according to God's design. Immediately after the Fall, dramatic changes occurred, none of them good. Peace, pleasure, and progress were no longer standard fare. They were replaced by strife, toil, and decline. Man became his own worst enemy. Endowed with tremendous capacity for good, he began using his abilities for self-gratification, trying desperately to fill the void within. In the process, he lost sight of what was truly needed—

to restore the lost relationship with God. So God pursued a plan whereby we would be . . .

Restored to God

In order to reach those who had been created in His image, God came to earth in their image. Jesus Christ, God's Son in flesh, came to earth. He lived a perfect life, which man could no longer do. He walked in total submission to the Father, which man had rejected. He taught about the truly important things in life, which man had forgotten. He died to pay the penalty for man's offenses, rose from the dead to gain victory over the forces of sin and death, and invited all to return to God and become His children. Many have. Others have not.

Let me stop at this point and talk to those who have not. The pursuit of satisfaction in life is futile apart from relationship with God. The void is caused by a missing relationship—a relationship you were created to enjoy. Take a moment now and find rest. Talk to God. Invite Jesus Christ to become Lord of your life. He will do for you what you can't do for yourself. Because everyone who trusts Him becomes . . .

A New Creature

The moment we accept our restored relationship with God, we are given a fresh start in life. We are even given a new identity. We change from God's enemy to God's friend. We change from a child of Satan to a child of God. Satan can no longer claim control over our lives when Jesus Christ takes the throne of our hearts. When the Lord takes over, He makes us completely new!

The Scriptures make several powerful statements about what occurs when we believe. If you want to improve your sense of identity, ponder this list describing those who have trusted Christ. From God's perspective, we become . . .

A child of God (John 1:12).
Christ's friend (John 15:15).
Chosen and appointed by Christ to bear His fruit (John 15:16).
Joint heir with Christ, sharing His inheritance with Him
(Romans 8:17).

Filled with God's Spirit and life (1 Corinthians 3:16; 6:19).

A member of Christ's Body (1 Corinthians 12:27; Ephesians 5:30).

A saint (Ephesians 1:1; Philippians 1:1).

God's workmanship—His handiwork—born anew in Christ to do His work (Ephesians 2:10).

A citizen of heaven (Philippians 3:20).

Chosen of God, holy and dearly loved (Colossians 3:12).

A son of light and not of darkness (1 Thessalonians 5:5).

A member of a chosen race, a royal priesthood, a holy nation (1 Peter 2:9–10).

THE ENEMY'S LIES

I can hear it now. "But I've been a Christian for years, and I don't feel like I'm any of those things. How can I be all of those things and still feel so miserable?"

Even though Satan has no formal authority over our lives, he still has a few tricks up his deceptive sleeve. If he can't have our soul, the next best thing is to rob us of our joy. (Joyful Christians really bug him!) One of the best ways to undermine our joy is to confuse our identity—to get us to believe lies about ourselves. Lies like . . .

"If you were as attractive as she is, others would like you better."

"You don't measure up. You're unworthy!"

"You only go around once, so live it up!"

"If you get that promotion, you'll finally feel good about yourself."

"If God really loves you, He'll give you what you want."

When we accept the lies, we live accordingly. You see, what we believe to be true has a direct impact upon our behavior, whether or not those beliefs are consistent with reality. Satan understands this principle all too well. Remember, he is the Father of Lies, and he knows his business.

In the first chapter I stated that the best way to make a man miserable is to confuse his definition of happiness. This is precisely what has happened. To one degree or another, we have all been brainwashed—believing ourselves to be worthless, like Sarah, a victim, like Paul, all alone, like Tammy, the center of the universe, like Bill, or some other falsity. Lies undermine our sense of identity. And

THE IMPACT OF IDENTITY

because our identity is misplaced, our actions follow suit. We begin to seek satisfaction in things that can never give it—material possessions, status, beauty, or whatever.

As Christians, we have access to lasting joy and fulfillment. But we often abandon the real thing for cheap imitations. C. S. Lewis described our dilemma well.

> If I find in myself a desire which no experience in this world can satisfy, the most probable explanation is that I was made for another world. If none of my earthly pleasures satisfy it, that does not prove that the universe is a fraud. Probably earthly pleasures were never meant to satisfy it, but only to arouse it, to suggest the real thing. If that is so, I must take care, on the one hand, never to despise, or be unthankful for, these earthly blessings, and on the other, never to mistake them for the something else of which they are only a kind of copy, or echo, or mirage. I must keep alive in myself the desire for my true country, which I shall not find till after death; I must never let it get snowed under or turned aside; I must make it the main object of life to press on to that other country and to help others to do the same.[2]

As Lewis suggests, the reason we can't find satisfaction in this life is that we miss step one. Before we can enjoy what we have, we must establish who we are. Unfortunately we often place our identity in our job, our house, our looks, or any number of temporal badges. The inevitable result? Discontentment. For this reason, it is important that we actively focus on the truth of who we are in Christ instead of believing the lies that undermine our joy. (For a better understanding of how Satan's lies can undermine our sense of identity, I strongly recommend the book *Victory Over the Darkness* by one of my former seminary professors, Dr. Neil Anderson.)

THE ANSWER

Let's go back to the shopping mall. According to the accurate "you are here" marker on the map, we were made in God's image with a built-in need and capacity for relationship with Him. Once that relationship is established, we have access to a lasting satisfaction that only He can provide.

Notice I said we *have access to* lasting satisfaction. I did not say we will always experience it. Filling the void within is only the first step on the road to contentment. Becoming a Christian no more guarantees perpetual contentment than it does trouble-free living. It does, however, provide us with the right map and an understanding of who we are, what we need, and where we can find it.

Getting Personal

Has your sense of identity depended on a good job, an attractive body, a large house, a fancy car, or any other temporal thing? Have you identified the spiritual roots of your discontentment? Have you intentionally defined who you are and what you need so you can actively pursue that which will satisfy? If you haven't yet done so, establish a relationship with God and allow Him to mold your identity into the one you were born to wear.

NOTE

1. C. S. Lewis, *Mere Christianity* (New York: Macmillan, 1952), 54.
2. Ibid., 120.

Chapter Seven

THE POWER OF PERSPECTIVE

Outlook determines outcome. Warren Wiersbe

Remember the Christmas classic, "It's a Wonderful Life"? The angel Clarence had been assigned to help George Bailey overcome his depression and give him a reason to press on. How did he do it? By fulfilling George's wish to have never been born and showing him what things would be like. George better understood the tremendous impact his life had on others for good by seeing all the bad that would have transpired without his influence. He saw his life for what it was, a splendid thing.

In the end, George returned to the same crummy circumstances with excitement and joyful anticipation. What was different? One very important thing—his perspective. Rather than viewing his predicament as a reason to throw in the towel, he realized it was merely an obstacle on the road of an otherwise wonderful life. He had come face to face with the possibility of losing everything he cherished, and it made a profound impact on his outlook. By simply changing his perspective on the circumstances of his life, George Bailey went from the valley of despair to the top of the mountain overnight.

How we view our circumstances dictates how we react to them. Our perspective can make the difference between viewing difficulty as a roadblock to success or as an opportunity for growth. It will determine whether we see life as a trial to endure or a party to enjoy. Depending upon our perspective, negative childhood experiences can become a lingering pain from our past or a foundation upon which to build a great future. Present circumstances can be seen as stumbling blocks or stepping stones, obstacles or opportunities. As George Bailey discovered, it all depends on our perspective. When we develop a healthy outlook on life in general, our circumstances no longer dictate our level of joy. Indeed, outlook does determine outcome.

A NEW POINT OF VIEW

One day a man who took great pride in his lawn suddenly found himself with a healthy crop of dandelions. He tried every conceivable method he knew to get rid of them, but nothing worked. Finally, he decided to write to the Department of Agriculture. He figured that if anyone knew how to deal with this problem, they would. After describing all his efforts to date, he closed the letter with the question, "What should I do now?" In due course came their reply—"We suggest you learn to live with them!"

There comes a point in life when we must learn to accept that which cannot be changed—when we must stop our futile striving to make life perfect. We need a new point of view—one that helps us maintain our priorities and our sanity.

Most of us fall into one of two extremes when it comes to discontentment. Both are the result of an unhealthy perspective on the circumstances of life. In the first category are those who perceive themselves as perpetual victims, always getting the short end of life's stick. These folks can't be content because things aren't right. They seek justice by demanding more, and they fully expect life to adapt to their desires. They feel they are entitled to something better. Needless to say, they are usually disappointed by the realities of life and quickly enter a state of passive disillusionment.

The second category includes those who are driven to achieve. They never relax because there is too much more to accomplish. There is always another mountain to climb or kingdom to conquer. We often describe these folks as high achievers. Unfortunately, the unrelenting drive for more keeps them from enjoying what they gain. They honestly believe that contentment will come as soon as the next goal is attained. But it never does.

Until we learn to accept the fact that we cannot eliminate or control the proverbial dandelions of life, we will never stop striving. An amazing thing transpires, however, when we develop a healthy perspective on our circumstances. We gain a calm confidence—an ability to rise above the details of life and observe them from a new point of view. No longer trapped in the quagmire of petty concerns, we begin living at a different level. The result, though not the goal, is contentment. We suddenly become comfortable with life as it is, rather than worry ourselves over how it should be.

If outlook determines outcome, how do we develop a perspective that will foster contentment? The secret is gaining the calm confidence that grows out of a healthy perspective on life. In order to gain this outlook, however, we must accept several important truths.

First, we must recognize that we cannot control our own fate. No matter how hard we try or how intensely we wish, it just is not within our power to control every circumstance or manipulate every outcome to fulfill our expectations. None of us is the master of his own destiny. All of us have limited influence and incomplete understanding. Sooner or later, we must all come to grips with the reality that we aren't God. So, the first step toward a healthy perspective on life is a healthy dose of humility—something none of us wants, but all of us need.

Second, we must rest in the truth of God's sovereign control over everything. Since we are not in control, we may as well stop trying so hard. There is a quiet rest which comes when we accept the fact that God is sovereign and we are not. It is foolish to cling so tightly to the reins of our lives when His loving hand has been guiding all along.

Finally, we must trade our expectations for God's plan. If God knows what is best, is it not likely that He will do what is best? If we want to foster true contentment, we must be willing to trust the one who has our best interest in mind. When we sacrifice our expectations on the altar of trust, the calm confidence of reliance replaces the anxiety of discontent.

THE KING WHO WOULD BE GOD

All of us must come to terms with our limitations. Often it becomes necessary to learn humility the hard way. Take Nebuchadnezzar, for example. He was the king of Babylon during its glory years. After conquering much of the known world, including Jerusalem, he was the leader of the most powerful and influential kingdom on earth. He was top banana, king of the hill, big man on campus. But he was not content. In fact, since ruling of the known world wasn't enough to satisfy his oversized ego, he decided to step up into a bigger role. He wanted to be God.

King Nebuchadnezzar was a very powerful man. No one in his right mind bucked Nebuchadnezzar's orders. No one, that is, except a few pesky Jews who had been transplanted from their homeland to serve in Nebuchadnezzar's court. Their Hebrew names were Daniel, Hananiah, Mishael, and Azariah—but they were given Babylonian names to help them better blend in with the crowd. It didn't work. They refused to blend.

Several incidents occurred which made these four guys stick out like a sore thumb—Nebuchadnezzar's thumb to be precise. First, they refused to eat the non-kosher foods provided by the king's guard. Second, one of them was able to interpret the king's prophetic dream after a failed attempt by all the other wise guys in town. Third, three of them were caught refusing to worship an image that had been built in honor of Nebuchadnezzar, despite a direct order. This particular incident really upset the king—something it wasn't in one's best interest to do. In fact, they were thrown into a burning furnace as punishment for blatant insubordination. Not to worry, though. They survived unscathed. God worked a miracle on their behalf, and it scared Nebuchadnezzar silly. So much so that he suddenly got religion. Let's pick up the story at the point where Shadrach, Meshach, and Abednego (as the Babylonians called them) are walking about in the fire unharmed.

> So Shadrach, Meshach and Abednego came out of the fire, and the satraps, prefects, governors and royal advisers crowded around them. They saw that the fire had not harmed their bodies, nor was a hair of their heads singed; their robes were not scorched, and there was no

114

smell of fire on them. Then Nebuchadnezzar said, "Praise be to the God of Shadrach, Meshach and Abednego, who has sent his angel and rescued his servants! They trusted in him and defied the king's command and were willing to give up their lives rather than serve or worship any god except their own God." (Daniel 3:26–28)

Not only did Nebuchadnezzar suddenly find religion, he decided to do God a big favor—he mandated reverence and respect for the Hebrew God. He even attached some pretty stiff penalties for those who might disagree: "I decree that the people of any nation or language who say anything against the God of Shadrach, Meshach and Abednego be cut into pieces and their houses be turned into piles of rubble, for no other god can save in this way" (Daniel 3:29).

A true convert, right? Wrong. Nebuchadnezzar did what any self-respecting king would do in such a frightful situation. He made a law that he hoped would appease God's anger. He had not learned true humility. In fact, one year later God found it necessary to teach him the humility lesson all over again. You see, Nebuchadnezzar had been on top for so long, he began to believe his own press. He was quite impressed with himself and with all he had accomplished. In short, he saw himself as God.

Twelve months later, as the king was walking on the roof of the royal palace of Babylon, he said, "Is not this the great Babylon I have built as the royal residence, by my mighty power and for the glory of my majesty?" (Daniel 4:29–30)

Right in the middle of his self-admiration dissertation, God interrupted Nebuchadnezzar to announce the method by which he would bring perspective back in line with reality.

The words were still on his lips when a voice came from heaven, "This is what is decreed for you, King Nebuchadnezzar: Your royal authority has been taken from you. You will be driven away from people and will live with the wild animals; you will eat grass like cattle. Seven times will pass by for you until you acknowledge that the Most High is sovereign over the kingdoms of men and gives them to anyone he wishes." Immediately what had been said about Nebuchadnezzar was fulfilled. He was driven away from people and ate grass like cattle. His body was drenched with the dew of heaven until his hair grew like the feathers of an eagle and his nails like the claws of a bird. (Daniel 4:31–33)

From all appearances, Nebuchadnezzar had a severe nervous breakdown—totally losing touch with reality. He came face to face with his own inadequacy and was confronted with the truth of God's sovereignty. It took a complete break with reality for Nebuchadnezzar to learn what reality is all about. And this time, he learned the lesson well. Let's peek at his diary for a firsthand summary of the results.

> At the end of that time, I, Nebuchadnezzar, raised my eyes toward heaven, and my sanity was restored. Then I praised the Most High; I honored and glorified him who lives forever. . . . At the same time that my sanity was restored, my honor and splendor were returned to me for the glory of my kingdom. My advisers and nobles sought me out, and I was restored to my throne and became even greater than before. Now I, Nebuchadnezzar, praise and exalt and glorify the King of heaven, because everything he does is right and all his ways are just. And those who walk in pride he is able to humble. (Daniel 4:34, 36–37)

Although he did it the hard way, Nebuchadnezzar ultimately acknowledged the truth of God's sovereign control over everything. But in order to do so, he first had to confront his own limitations. The end result was a man more equipped to sit on the throne, and a man no longer prone to make himself God.

MAKING OURSELVES GOD

None of us will ever become a world ruler like Nebuchadnezzar. But his status does not make him unique. Though he may have had more opportunity to demonstrate a warped perspective, his basic problem was no different than that of any of us. His experience serves as an extreme example of what happens when a man makes himself God. And whether we will admit it or not, all of us fall into the same trap from time to time.

We make ourselves God when we insist that circumstances cooperate with our game plan. We make ourselves God when we covet what others possess. We make ourselves God when we envy another person's looks, status, wealth, mate, upbringing, job, lifestyle, or popularity. We make ourselves God when we perceive our own efforts to be the sole source of our success. Like Nebuchadnezzar, we look around at the good things we've attained, congratulate ourselves on a job well done, and look for the next kingdom to conquer. Regardless of the specific expression of our pride, we make ourselves God every time we take the reins of control out of His hands and attempt to guide life toward our own ends. We reject His sovereign authority and make ourselves the God of our own lives. The cause and the outcome are the same—discontentment.

More often than not, discontentment grows out of an unwillingness to trust God with our circumstances. We cling tightly to our own vision of how life should be, refusing to let go at any cost. Rather than resting in the knowledge of God's control and traveling with a gentle grip on a lightly-packed suitcase, we resist the inevitable. Unfortunately, the price we pay may be a life of missed joys and needless strife. Ultimately, we will reach a point where reality must pry our expectations loose from our firm grip—leaving nothing but disillusionment and bitterness as a legacy to our stubborn resolve.

A. W. Tozer described God's sovereignty using the analogy of an ocean liner leaving New York bound for Liverpool. The ship's captain has been given the responsibility, and authority, to navigate the ship to its predetermined destination. On board the ship are hundreds of passengers, all free to roam about as they wish. They can enjoy the journey without concerning themselves over the ship's ultimate destination. The captain has things well in control, and nothing anyone may say or do will change his actions. He knows the way, and he is responsible for the ship's safe and timely arrival to a predetermined port in Liverpool.[1] How foolish it would be for the passengers to spend the entire journey worrying about every shifting wind or turn of the rudder. What good would it do to become anxious over that which they have no influence or understanding? And yet, that is precisely what we do when we concern ourselves over those things that only God has the power to change.

As Christians, we know that God is in control and that He has our ultimate best interest in mind. But we have trouble transferring that abstract truth into the practical day to day of life. If we truly believed our rhetoric, the calm confidence of trusting God's plan for our lives would overshadow the disappointment of unmet expectations. We would find the ability to rise above our circumstances, good or bad, and rest in the knowledge of God's ultimate control over our destination. It would no longer matter whether we have that nicer home, better job, or perfect mate. If we truly trusted God's plan, we could stop worrying and enjoy the journey. Once we take ourselves out of His role, our expectations will fall in line. Then we can truly experience the rest of contentment and the freedom of letting God be God.

God's Wonderful Plan

Frank entered the Christian life as an adult, through the work of a large evangelistic missions organization. Its literature taught him about four spiritual laws, the first of which said that God loved him and had a wonderful plan for his life. This sounded appealing to Frank because his life thus far had been anything but wonderful. Prior to his conversion, Frank had been part of the drug culture and was ruled by the quest for self-gratification. The trouble was, it was quickly leading him down a path to self-destruction. Frank fully embraced what Christ had to offer. Grateful that he had been saved from a rather miserable experience, Frank dedicated his life to full-time Christian service. He could hardly wait to discover the wonderful plan God had for him.

Frank was confident that he knew at least part of God's plan for his life due to two passions that entered his heart shortly after becoming a believer. The first was the desire to go to the mission field and evangelize an entire country for Christ. Toward this end, Frank began working for a Christian ministry which promoted world missions. The second was the desire to marry a nice Christian girl and have lots of kids. He knew that marriage was ordained by God, and that children are a blessing from the Lord. Frank was certain that both desires would be fulfilled in his life as part of God's wonderful plan. Otherwise, why would He have put them in his heart?

Twenty years later, Frank is still single and still working for a Christian ministry in the States. He has never met the right girl, nor has he ever served on a foreign mission field. He struggles in his relationship with the Lord because he is disillusioned. "If God loves me and has a wonderful plan for my life," Frank wonders, "then why haven't the deep longings He gave me been fulfilled?"

Frank has had to reckon with the possibility that God's wonderful plan for our lives may not match our own idea of what that plan should be. Many of us follow the Lord with an expectation that His plan for our lives will be the same as our own. We have trouble recognizing that we are not the center of God's universe. It may be that His plan is bigger, and better, than our specific desires. Or it may be our personal lack of initiative that keeps God from using us. Frank discovered that technical details such as raising support are part of the process of traveling to the mission field, and they require a lot of effort.

The Altar of Trust

One of the most liberating experiences of life is when we sacrifice our expectations on the altar of trust—when we finally release those things which have prevented us from enjoying the freedom of contentment. Unfortunately, few of us ever reach this place of rest because it requires a very difficult step. We must allow trust in God's plan to overshadow our own dreams and desires.

Abraham was confronted with the choice between holding onto that which he most cherished or sacrificing it on the altar of trust. In his case, it was a literal sacrifice on a real altar. God asked Abraham to take his son Isaac up to the mountains and take his son's life as a burnt offering. Isaac had been born to Abraham and Sarah in their old age in fulfillment of a promise that Abraham's descendants would become a great nation. Since he was their only child, Isaac embodied all of Abraham's hopes and dreams. So this sacrifice meant more than the death of a beloved child. It also represented the death of Abraham's expectations. If there was one time Abraham could have questioned God's better judgment, this was it. But he didn't. He proceeded to follow the Lord's instructions, releasing his expectations in the process.

> When they reached the place God had told him about, Abraham built an altar there and arranged the wood on it. He bound his son Isaac and laid him on the altar, on top of the wood. Then he reached out his hand and took the knife to slay his son. (Genesis 22:9–10)

I have often wondered what was going through Abraham's mind at this point, not to mention Isaac's. In this moment of crisis, Abraham had the calm confidence to proceed with the most difficult sacrifice of his life. How could he carry out such an awful command? He had developed a perspective which allowed him to trust. He knew God on a personal level, and he had confidence that everything would work for the best. And that, in a nutshell, is what the faith-walk is all about. In fact, a tribute to this obedient act of Abraham is posted in what has been commonly called the New Testament Hall of Faith: "By faith Abraham, when God tested him, offered Isaac as a sacrifice. He who had received the promises was about to sacrifice his one and only son, even though God had said to him, 'It is through Isaac that your offspring will be reckoned.' Abraham reasoned that God could raise the dead, and figuratively speaking, he did receive Isaac back from death" (Hebrews 11:17–19). In essence, Abraham had more confidence in God's ultimate control over the situation than in his own understanding of it. And God rewarded his faith as a result. Let's return to the story at the point when Abraham was lowering the knife to Isaac's throat.

> But the angel of the Lord called out to him from heaven, "Abraham! Abraham! . . . Do not lay a hand on the boy," he said. "Do not do anything to him. Now I know that you fear God, because you have not withheld from me your son, your only son." . . . The angel of the Lord called to Abraham from heaven a second time and said, "I swear by myself, declares the Lord, that because you have done this and have not withheld your son, your only son, I will surely bless you and make your descendants as numerous as the stars in the sky and as the sand on the seashore. Your descendants will take possession of the cities of their enemies, and through your offspring all nations on earth will be blessed, because you have obeyed me." (Genesis 22:11–12, 15–18)

Abraham approached the altar of trust and sacrificed his most cherished expectation on it. As a result, he could rest in the knowledge that God would accomplish greater things than he could ever have imagined. By trusting the one who holds tomorrow, Abraham caught a glimpse of the future. He experienced what has been promised to all believers: "And we know that in all things God works for the good of those who love him, who have been called according to his purpose" (Romans 8:28).

It is important to note that God did not want Isaac's life; He wanted Abraham's trust. In like manner, we may not need to sacrifice the things we expect, just the expectations themselves. Abraham's dream became a reality, but only after he was willing to give it up. We may well receive all the things we expect in life, but we can only enjoy them when we stop demanding them. As Abraham discovered, releasing our expectations and trusting God's plan for our lives can open the door for Him to give us the joy we want and the rest we need. Even when the details vary from our own dreams, His plan is best.

How does Karen find fulfillment when her plans to marry and have children never become a reality? By sacrificing her expectations on the altar of trust. How does Jane come to terms with the fact that a homemaker's daily grind will never match her "happily ever after" fantasy? By sacrificing her expectations on the altar of trust. How does Mark remain motivated when he is overlooked for promotion—again? By sacrificing his expectations on the altar of trust. Whatever the specific source of disappointment, the solution is the same. We must take the Lord's extended hand and trust Him to lead us. But before we can place our hand in His, we must stop clutching so tightly to our expectations. Letting go may be painful. But it is not nearly as painful as holding on.

Trust in the Tough Times

The Old Testament book of Job tells the story of a remarkable man who demonstrated contentment in both the good times and the tough times thanks to his perspective on the circumstances of life. Job was a very wealthy, influential man in his day. He was also a very generous and caring individual. He had managed to achieve both financial wealth and depth of character, making him one of God's prize pupils. So much so that the story opens with the Lord bragging on Job's life to Satan:

> The Lord said to Satan, "Have you considered my servant Job? There is no one on earth like him; he is blameless and upright, a man who fears God and shuns evil." "Does Job fear God for nothing?" Satan replied. "Have you not put a hedge around him and his household and everything he has? You have blessed the work of his hands, so that his

flocks and herds are spread throughout the land. But stretch out your hand and strike everything he has, and he will surely curse you to your face." (Job 1:8–11)

Satan's logic seems reasonable enough. It is easy to trust God, and find contentment, when we have everything we want. But take the good things away and see what happens. In this case, the Lord allowed Satan to wreak havoc in Job's life. He lost all his material wealth and all his children in the same day. What was his response to the loss?

At this, Job got up and tore his robe and shaved his head. Then he fell to the ground in worship and said: "Naked I came from my mother's womb, and naked I will depart. The Lord gave and the Lord has taken away; may the name of the Lord be praised." (Job 1:20–21)

Sure, he grieved. But he also demonstrated the power of perspective by falling to his knees and praising God in the midst of his tragedy. Job recognized that God is ultimately in control, even in the bad times. He was able to endure and accept awful circumstances because he let God be God. As a result, Job was content in both the good and the bad of life.

A short time later, God allowed Satan to inflict a very painful disease upon Job's body. If he couldn't get Job to break under the strain of catastrophic loss, maybe he could get him with physical illness. Well, Satan didn't break Job, but he did break Job's wife.

His wife said to him, "Are you still holding on to your integrity? Curse God and die!" He replied, "You are talking like a foolish woman. Shall we accept good from God, and not trouble?" In all this, Job did not sin in what he said. (Job 2:9–10)

When we understand God's sovereign right to do as He wishes, it does something to our perspective on the circumstances of life— as Job demonstrated in the midst of a situation far worse than any of us is likely to endure. One day he had all the money he could want, a healthy body, and a happy family. The next day he was a penniless, sickly man with a bitter wife. Yet his trust was as strong, or stronger, in the tough times. His secret? Perspective. He had sacrificed his expectations on the altar of trust.

After spending some time with friends, all of whom were convinced that Job had done something wrong to deserve his plight, Job faced understandable discouragement. Perhaps worse than the pain and loss he felt was the silence from heaven. He trusted God, and he knew that he had done nothing to deserve these circumstances. But God didn't seem to care enough to explain why. Job wanted answers. What God gave him, instead, were questions.

> Brace yourself like a man; I will question you, and you shall answer me. Where were you when I laid the earth's foundation? Tell me, if you understand. Who marked off its dimensions? Surely you know! . . . Have you ever given orders to the morning, or shown the dawn its place? . . . Have the gates of death been shown to you? . . . Have you comprehended the vast expanses of the earth? Tell me, if you know all this. . . . Can you bring forth the constellations in their seasons? Or lead out the Bear with its cubs? Do you know the laws of the heavens? Can you set up God's dominion over the earth? . . . Who endowed the heart with wisdom or gave understanding to the mind? Will the one who contends with the Almighty correct him? Let him who accuses God answer him! (Job 38:2–5, 12, 17–18, 32–33, 36; 39:2)

At first pass, the Lord seems to be placing a cruel burden upon Job's shoulders. After all, he only wanted to know why life had fallen apart. Not only did his question remain unanswered, God responded in a manner that would seem to drive Job further into despair. On the contrary. You see, what Job *wanted* were answers. But what Job *needed* was relationship. He needed to be reminded, once again, that God was in control. And when his trust in the God of all power and goodness was reaffirmed, Job regained the perspective he needed to cope with the hardships of life.

Job was ultimately restored to health, wealth, and ten more kids. But the lesson grows out of the difficult trial, not the happy ending. When we face the pain of unmet expectations and the tough times life can bring, what we need is renewed perspective. We need to be reminded that God is in control and He knows best. We may or may not face a happy ending. But like Job, we can experience contentment in the midst of good or bad if our life is grounded in the powerful truth of God's sovereignty.

A Calm Confidence

Once we learn to maintain a perspective of trust, we can finally enter a state of rest. This perspective changed Nebuchadnezzar from an arrogant, greedy dictator into a humble, contented king who recognized God's ultimate authority. This perspective allowed Abraham to sacrifice what he most wanted in order to gain what he most needed. This perspective gave three young Jews the courage to do what was right despite the threat of a blazing furnace. This perspective enabled Job to trust God's plan in the midst of severe loss and suffering. This perspective led an imprisoned apostle Paul to say, "I have learned to be content in every situation." By trusting the God who controls everything, these men were able to rise above their circumstances and rest in the calm confidence of contented living. And so can we.

Every parent has dreams of what his or her children can become. Sometimes those dreams come true, and sometimes they are shattered into nightmarish fragments. Some parents can identify with the Old Testament patriarch Job, whose ten children were killed in one day. What are parents' choices when dreams die or are derailed along with their children? When a long-awaited child is born with handicaps, when a teenager is killed by a drunk driver, when a son is murdered or imprisoned, when a young unmarried daughter becomes pregnant? It's easy to speak of trust when times are easy. But in the hard times, the answers are no easier than the questions. Yet trust in God, though hardest under such circumstances, can also be ultimately truest then.

Perhaps the most effective way we can foster a spirit of trust, and the resulting sense of contentment, is to read and reread those passages of Scripture that highlight the truth of God's sovereign control over the details of life. Reminding ourselves that He is captain of the ship helps us maintain a healthy perspective on the circumstances of life. I believe a primary reason that the Bible repeatedly highlights the truth of God's greatness is to calm our anxious spirits and free us from the fear of uncertainty—both of which breed discontentment. As someone has said, we need not be afraid to trust an unknown future to an all-knowing God.

The psalmist expresses well just how much God does know about each of us:

> O Lord, you have searched me and you know me. You know when I sit and when I rise; you perceive my thoughts from afar. You discern my going out and my lying down; you are familiar with all my ways. Before a word is on my tongue you know it completely, O Lord. . . . For you created my inmost being; you knit me together in my mother's womb. I praise you because I am fearfully and wonderfully made; your works are wonderful, I know that full well. My frame was not hidden from you when I was made in the secret place. When I was woven together in the depths of the earth, your eyes saw my unformed body. All the days ordained for me were written in your book before one of them came to be. (Psalm 139:1–4, 13–16)

When we truly understand and embrace the reality of God's ultimate control, we can stop worrying about the ship's destination. The end result is a calm confidence that brings rest, and contentment, to our frantic lives.

Getting Personal

H ave you learned to rest in the knowledge of God's ultimate control over the details of life? Have you sacrificed your expectations on the altar of trust? He knows the destination, and He is steering the ship. How about simply letting God be God, and start enjoying the journey?

NOTE

1. A. W. Tozer, *The Knowledge of the Holy* (San Francisco: HarperSanFrancisco, 1992), 174.

Chapter Eight

THE CURSE
OF COMPARISON

If you compare yourself with others, you may become bitter or vain, for always there will be greater and lesser persons than yourself. Max Ehrman

I have found that my level of contentment varies from day to day depending upon which way I drive to work in the morning. If I drive through the rich part of town, I find myself wanting more than I have. If I drive through the poor part of town, I consider myself wealthy. I guess I should always drive through the poor part of town, right? Wrong. The problem is not that I am comparing my status to the wrong group, but that I am comparing it at all.

The quickest way to undermine contentment is to compare ourselves to others. We will always find someone who has it better than we do, and we will always find someone who has it worse. Depending on our point of comparison, we will become bitter or vain. In both instances the root problem is the same—we place our focus in the wrong place. We become victims to the curse of comparison.

Comparisons come in many shapes and sizes. There are good and bad comparisons. A good comparison fosters healthy competition in the athletic, academic, or business setting. A bad comparison causes us to view our present situation as inadequate or inferior. More often than not, unfortunately, we tend toward the latter.

A person can't live in modern society without being bombarded by reminders of what he lacks. Movies and television make fantasy appear to be reality—a reality far more exciting than your ho-hum existence. The check-out stand at the grocery store displays magazine covers that glamorize the rich and the beautiful—another reminder that you don't measure up. The multi-billion-dollar advertising industry is built around one primary objective—making you feel inadequate. Television commercials, billboards, magazine ads, direct mail promotions, and fashion displays are all designed to help you compare yourself to others and convince you that you need something more before you can be happy. Unfortunately, it works all too well. They don't sell us products. They sell us discontentment.

ONE OF GOD'S TOP TEN

At the root of most discontentment is the desire for something we don't currently possess. Unsatisfied with life as it is, we want something more. Usually, someone else has the something we want —a nicer home, a newer car, a better job, a healthier body, a more attractive mate (or any mate at all). Whatever the specific point of comparison, the result is envy—and the violation of a very important command given to Moses on Mount Sinai. "You shall not covet your neighbor's house. You shall not covet your neighbor's wife, or his manservant or maidservant, his ox or donkey, or anything that belongs to your neighbor" (Exodus 20:17).

That's right, the issue of contentment is addressed in God's top ten. It made it onto the list alongside the biggies like murder, theft, and adultery. Surprised?

At first glance the covet commandment seems overrated. I mean, what's the big deal? Comparing and desiring what others have isn't like murder or theft. So why did the Lord make such an issue over it? I'll tell you why. Because of the impact it has upon our life choices and attitudes. More than anything else, covetousness can motivate warped priorities. And when our priorities are wrong, our actions will follow suit.

Like most of the laws and commandments listed in the Bible, it is not always easy to heed the caution against covetousness. It is so natural to desire the things we see others enjoying. The covet factor is such a powerful force because we all have a natural propensity toward envy. All of us inherited the tendency and live with the inevitable result—discontentment.

Consider your own experience. Do you have friends with a nicer home? Does visiting their abode make it difficult to remain content with your own? What about your job? Do you find it tough to be happy for someone who got the promotion you wanted? Or how about the girl who just got engaged to a great guy while you can't even get a date—are you tempted to hate her? If you said yes to any of these questions, you are quite normal—and in violation of the tenth commandment. God gave the caution against coveting such prominent billing precisely because it is such a natural part of our lives. But it is also very damaging, and we must learn to deal with it before it poisons our whole existence.

If you were exposed to any form of media during the 1994 winter Olympics, you'll remember the constant focus upon two people— Tonya Harding and Nancy Kerrigan. It seems that Tonya Harding was intensely jealous of Nancy's success, to the point that she and her former husband consorted to do something about it. According to later investigations, Tonya conspired an attack on Nancy in order to keep her out of competition. In the end, Nancy wound up with an Olympic medal and was considered a national hero for overcoming a painful obstacle to obtain victory. Tonya, on the other hand, became a national symbol of shame and a reminder of what can happen when we allow comparison to foster jealousy and envy.

During the 1930s a man named Hitler led an entire nation to provoke one of the most destructive and evil conflicts the world has ever known. How did he do it? By convincing the German people that they deserved better than they had. They proceeded to demand it, then seize it, then kill to get it.

Today, thousands will make themselves miserable by comparing their lives and possessions with those around them. They will lose sight of the good things because they covet the apparently better things. Person by person, family by family, nation by nation, we ruin ourselves through the fine art of comparison. Is it any wonder that God cautioned us so strongly on this point? He knows all too well the kinds of individual and corporate evil comparisons can cause.

FROM A DISTANCE

Once upon a time there was a king named Dionysius who ruled the richest city in Sicily. He lived in a beautiful palace and possessed great wealth. He had many servants who waited on him day and night. Because Dionysius was so rich and powerful, many envied his good fortune—including his very good friend Damocles. Damocles repeatedly said to Dionysius, "How lucky you are! You have every-thing anyone could want. You must be the happiest man alive."

One day Dionysius became weary of such talk. "Do you really think I am happier than everyone else?" he asked Damocles.

"Of course you are," Damocles replied. "Just look at the great treasures you possess and the power you hold. You don't have a sin-gle worry. Life couldn't be any better."

"Perhaps you would like to change places with me," said Diony-sius.

"I couldn't do that," said Damocles. "But if I could only have your riches and your pleasures for one day, I should never want any greater happiness."

"Very well. You will trade places with me for one day."

The next day, Damocles was brought to the palace, and all the servants were instructed to treat him as their master. He wore the royal robes and the crown of gold. He sat at the royal table to be served rich foods in a fine setting. He lacked nothing that could give him pleasure that day. He had costly food and wine, obedient ser-vants, lovely flowers, rare perfumes, and delightful music. As he rested himself on the soft royal cushions, he considered himself the happi-est man alive.

"Ah, this is the life. I've never enjoyed myself as much," he thought.

Just then, while lifting the royal cup to his lips, he raised his eyes toward the ceiling. There was something dangling above him, almost touching his head. Damocles became very tense. The smile faded from his lips, and the color drained from his face. His hands began to tremble. He did not want any more food, wine, or music. He just wanted to leave the palace and get far away. You see, directly above his head hung a sword, held to the ceiling by only a single horsehair. Its blade glittered as it pointed right between his eyes. He started to leap to run, but he stopped himself. He was afraid that any sudden movement would cause the thin thread to snap, allowing the sword to plunge downward. He sat stiff and frightened in the chair.

"What is wrong, my friend?" asked Dionysius. "You seem to have lost your appetite."

"That sword! That sword!" whispered Damocles. "Don't you see it there above my head?"

"Of course I do," said Dionysius. "I see it there every day of my life. It always hangs over my head, and there is always the chance that something will cause it to fall. Perhaps one of my advisers will become jealous of my power and try to kill me. Or someone may spread lies about me, and turn the people against me. Maybe a neighboring kingdom will send an army to seize my throne. Or I could make an unwise decision that will bring my downfall. If you want to be a leader, you must be willing to accept the risks. You see, they come with the wealth and power."

"Yes, I do see," said Damocles. "I see that I was mistaken to envy you so. Please take your place back, and allow me to return to my own house."

For the rest of Damocles's life, he never again wanted to change places with the king. Not even for a moment.[1]

The lesson of Damocles's sword is clear. When we look upon the good fortune of another, we are only seeing his experience from a distance. Close up, we may gain an entirely different perspective. Comparison is folly because it is built upon partial truth. Once the whole picture becomes clear, envy may quickly fade.

CONSEQUENCES

There are countless direct and indirect consequences to the comparison game—none of them very good. Perhaps the most notable is the impact it can have on our perspective. As you'll recall from our discussion in chapter 8, maintaining a lasting sense of contentment depends on a healthy view of God's plan for our lives. Unfortunately, when we take our eyes off Him and look at those around us, we undermine the rest which grows out of simple trust.

Free at Last!

The people of ancient Israel were a fickle bunch. While living in the land of Egypt as slaves, they wanted freedom. Shortly after leaving Egypt as free men and women, they began complaining and asking Moses to take them back to Egypt. They had discovered that the greener grass of freedom was located over the septic tank of hard work and a limited menu. Slavery had been no picnic, but at least there was more than bread and water to satisfy their appetites.

Despite their grumbling, Moses didn't take them back to Egypt. After a forty-year detour, they entered the Promised Land. A land flowing with milk and honey was theirs. Freedom had never smelled so sweet. No more dusty travels, no more dry dinners, and no more taking orders from that Moses fellow. Finally in Canaan where they belonged, God's rule book in hand, they had judges to help them sort out right from wrong. They didn't need a demanding ruler to boss them around anymore. They were free from slavery, free from the trial of desert travels, and free from being under the thumb of the man Moses. Free at last.

It wasn't long before the people of Israel lost sight of God's hand in their lives—not to mention His rules for their lives. They began breaking the simple commands He had given, especially the one about serving other gods. They took themselves out from under His protective control. They worshiped idols, forgot about the Lord, and did evil. Enslaved to their own wicked passions, they spiraled downward—ultimately ending up in bondage to foreign powers.

It became necessary for God to bail out the people of Israel time and time again over the next several generations. The cycle was predictable. First, they would forget about God, falling into idolatry and evil. Second, the Lord allowed a foreign power to conquer them in order to get their attention. Third, they would call out to God for help. Finally, He would respond by sending a deliverer to redeem them. Some of the more famous heroes of this period include Gideon (the guy who defeated an army by blowing trumpets and smashing lamps) and Samson (the muscle man with a mindless attraction to Delilah).

Time after time they abandoned God. Time after time they asked Him for help. Time after time He rescued them—only to be forgotten again. And yet, the Lord remained faithful to Israel through it all. They couldn't ask for a better Sovereign. Or could they?

We Want a King

At this point in the drama of Jewish history the people of Israel looked around and noticed something significant. Every other nation of the world had something they didn't—a king. God had deliberately established Himself as their King (a theocracy) because He knew the problems associated with following a human king (a monarchy). But the people lost sight of the benefits as soon as they began comparing themselves to other nations. They wanted a physical king sitting on a real throne located in a royal palace in the midst of a capital city. Faith in God was hard to maintain. Trust in human royalty seemed better.

Samuel, God's spokesman, tried to talk the people out of establishing a human king. He explained the potential hardships that could follow—like a national draft, high taxes, the loss of personal independence, and the other burdens which go along with royal rule.

> But the people refused to listen to Samuel. "No!" they said. "We want a king over us. Then we will be like all the other nations, with a king to lead us and to go out before us and fight our battles." (1 Samuel 8:19-20)

Notice their motivation. They wanted to be like all the other nations. It wasn't that they felt abandoned by God or that the present system was a flop. It was plain old-fashioned envy. They wanted a human king because everyone else had one. The curse of comparison led them to usurp God's plan and set up a system that would ultimately lead to their national demise. As the Lord told Samuel, "It is not you they have rejected, but they have rejected me as their king" (1 Samuel 8:7).

This leads us to the first consequence of the comparison trap.

COMPARISON CONSEQUENCE #1: Comparisons lead us to desire what is popular rather than what is best.

Why do we do that? One minute we can be completely content with God's wonderful plan for our lives, and the next minute we are drooling over the latest gadget, fad, or fashion. If someone else has it, we want it too. Whether or not we can afford it, need it, like it, or know how to use it is beside the point. Many a foolish decision has been motivated by the desire for what is popular.

A healthy perspective can be quickly undermined by a glance to the right or left. We lose sight of what is best in favor of, well, anything else that comes along. Rather than enjoying the natural wealth of contentment, we make ourselves poor. And, like the people of Israel, we often reject God's good gifts along the way.

"Hey, What About Me?"

Picture this scene. My two young sons are sitting in front of the television set watching a big purple dinosaur sing silly songs. They are completely content with their present situation—no complaints, no worries. Suddenly, Mom walks over and quietly hands one of them a chocolate chip cookie. For a few moments the other doesn't notice what just happened. He's still completely content. But then, upon hearing the familiar sound of cookie consumption, he glances over at his brother. The scene now turns ugly. A child who was happy and satisfied only moments earlier is instantaneously changed into a sniveling, whining, discontent victim. "Hey, what about me?" "I want one too!" "That's not fair!"

Change scenes. You leave for work in the morning completely content with your life. You look great, feel great, and have it all. As you pull into the parking lot, you notice the cars on either side of your space. Both of them are very nice and very new. Suddenly, the six-year-old mode of transportation which just got you to work with no trouble becomes a "bucket of bolts" or a "pile of junk." Upon entering the office, you pass several secretaries—all of whom have perfect figures and cover-girl hair. Suddenly, you don't feel so attractive. As you begin your workday, you take your seat across from the director's office. He has it made. A great job, a huge salary, a healthy expense account, and from what you've heard, a very large home. Suddenly, the job you've worked so hard to attain doesn't pay enough or perk enough. Like my son eyeing his brother's cookie, your contented existence quickly sours—turning you into a sniveling, whining, discontent victim. "Hey, what about me?" "I want one too!" "Life's not fair!"

That's right, life isn't fair. We don't all receive the same level of opportunity or blessing in this life. Part of content living is learning to accept that reality. So we might as well stop our envious gaze at the cookie in someone else's hand and start enjoying what we've got.

Jesus told a story that dramatically illustrated how we sniveling humans tend to respond to the cookie scenario. Let's take a look at his words as found in Matthew 20.

> For the kingdom of heaven is like a landowner who went out early in the morning to hire men to work in his vineyard. He agreed to pay them a denarius for the day and sent them into his vineyard. About the third hour he went out and saw others standing in the marketplace doing nothing. He told them, "You also go and work in my vineyard, and I will pay you whatever is right." So they went. He went out again about the sixth hour and the ninth hour and did the same thing. About the eleventh hour he went out and found still others standing around. He asked them, "Why have you been standing here all day long doing nothing?" "Because no one has hired us," they answered. He said to them, "You also go and work in my vineyard." (vv. 1–7)

Jesus is illustrating a kingdom principle with a very common occurrence in an agrarian society—laborers waiting in the marketplace for someone to hire them for the day. A parallel for today might be a factory owner walking into the unemployment office and offering everyone a job. Note that the landowner in the story represents God. The workers were unemployed when the day began. Thanks to the landowner, they would now be earning a paycheck. Everyone should be happy, right? Wrong. Let's pick up the story as the final whistle blows.

> When evening came, the owner of the vineyard said to his foreman, "Call the workers and pay them their wages, beginning with the last ones hired and going on to the first." The workers who were hired about the eleventh hour came and each received a denarius. So when those came who were hired first, they expected to receive more. But each one of them also received a denarius. When they received it, they began to grumble against the landowner. "These men who were hired last worked only one hour," they said, "and you have made them equal to us who have borne the burden of the work and the heat of the day." (vv. 8–12)

They have a point. After working a twelve-hour shift in the hot sun, they received the same pay as the guys who strolled in late in the day and worked a mere sixty minutes. If anyone had a reason to cry foul, it would seem that these guys did. "Hey, what about me!" "Life's not fair!"

> But he answered one of them, "Friend, I am not being unfair to you. Didn't you agree to work for a denarius? Take your pay and go. I want to give the man who was hired last the same as I gave you. Don't I have the right to do what I want with my own money? Or are you envious because I am generous?"

Ouch! Good comeback, landowner. They did have an agreement that was honored on both sides. The owner did nothing wrong, dishonest, or sneaky. He paid them 100 percent of the agreed-upon wage. So why all the complaining? The landowner hit the nail on the head—"because I am generous." The workers weren't complaining because they had it so bad. They were complaining because some-one else had it better. Brother got a cookie and they didn't.

This leads us to the second consequence of the comparison trap.

COMPARISON CONSEQUENCE #2: When we focus on the blessings of others, we become ungrateful for our own blessings.

I believe Jesus is teaching the principle that God does not dole out blessings or opportunities equally in this life. Yet He never promised that He would. He said He would meet all our needs, not give us all our wants. Just as the landowner did what he wanted with his own money, the Lord does what He wants with His own blessings. We can either learn to live with that reality and be grateful for the good gifts He gives us, or we can resist it and become sniveling, whining, and discontent people.

It might be appropriate at this point to stop and pray a prayer.

Lord, help me to focus on the blessings You've given me, rather than the blessings You've given others. Keep me from becoming envious because You are generous. Don't let me rob myself of enjoying the good just because others may have it better. Thank You that I am no longer "unemployed," but have been blessed with many gifts from Your hand. Amen.

The Reunion Ruin

My wife and I attended her ten-year high-school reunion several years ago. She had been quite popular as a high school.senior. In fact, she was the homecoming queen. (Our marriage is proof positive that a high school nerd can end up with a homecoming queen!) As an outsider, it was fun to attend and observe. I only knew two people at the reunion—my wife's best friend Darcee and her husband, Karl. Neither Karl nor I had attended this school, so we just blended into the background and watched as the drama of nostalgic chatter, screams of recognition, and politely veiled shock played out before us.

An interesting dynamic occurred the minute these old friends got together. The subtle yet obvious comparison game began in full force. Conversations centered around such themes as marriage, children, career success, and financial status. Few who had been highly successful did any overt bragging. But the point was made wherever it could be conveniently slipped into the conversation.

Karl and I saw single women eyeing the married-with-children gang with envy. We observed the proud blue-collar worker deflate while chatting with the white-collar crowd. The homemaker felt inferior to the professional woman. The former cheerleader who had gained thirty pounds politely hated the former wallflower who had lost twenty. The divorced single mom no longer identified with her former best pal, now happily married to a successful architect. In short, nearly everyone seemed to leave the event feeling less satisfied with how his or her life had turned out than when he or she came. I'm sure many wondered why they had even bothered to attend.

It is easy to say that we should rest in God's plan for our lives. But it is often hard to do—especially when His plan for others seems so much better. The apostle Peter encountered these same feelings at a reunion of his own.

What About Him?

A few days after the death of Christ, Peter and the other disheartened disciples returned to their roots and went fishing. While they were in the boat, the resurrected Jesus appeared on the shore and called out to them. He instructed them to throw the net overboard—leading them directly to a mega catch. Peter knew immediately that it must be the Lord. So he jumped in the water and swam to meet Him.

They sat down together for breakfast. After they ate, Jesus asked the excited Peter what seemed like a simple question—"Do you love Me?" But there was more to the question than it seemed on the surface. If you'll recall, Peter had denied the Lord three times a few days earlier after proclaiming his never-dying loyalty. Peter answered without hesitation. "Yes, Lord. You know that I love You."

"Feed My lambs," Jesus responded. Then He asked again, "Do you truly love Me?"

Peter answered again. "Yes, Lord. You know that I love You."

"Take care of My sheep," He instructed, just before asking again, "Do you love Me?"

This time it hit home with Peter. Through his hurt, Peter responded. "Lord, You know all things; You know that I love You."

"Feed My sheep." Then Jesus said something very interesting. "I tell you the truth, when you were a child you dressed yourself and went where you wanted; but when you are old you will stretch out your hands, and someone else will dress you and lead you where you do not want to go."

What does that mean? John 21:19 tells us that Jesus said this to indicate the kind of death by which Peter would glorify God. Then He said to him, "Follow Me!"

Tradition tells us that Peter died by being crucified upside down. At the very least we know that he suffered in his death for the cause of Christ.

Having been told of God's plan for his life, Peter immediately seeks to compare his future lot to the others. He spots John. "Lord, what about him?"

Jesus answered, "If I want him to remain alive until I return, what is that to you? *You* must follow Me." To paraphrase, "What happens to him is none of your business, Peter. I told you to follow Me!"

Peter allowed the comparison game to divert his attention from God's plan for his life. As a result, Jesus had to remind him to mind his own business—which highlights our third comparison consequence.

COMPARISON CONSEQUENCE #3: Focusing on God's plan for others can cause us to neglect His plan for us.

"But their lives seem so much more exciting, interesting, comfortable, pleasant, fair, etc." Maybe they do. But those are their lives, not yours. God's plan for others may look nothing like His plan for you. Accept it, deal with it, mind your own business, and move on. You are responsible to pursue and make the most of the opportunities and challenges confronting *you,* not those confronting the guy next door. Who knows? If we stopped wasting so much time and energy staring at the lives of others, we might have more left to make ours more profitable, meaningful, and enjoyable.

| *Getting Personal* . . . .

H ave you been allowing the comparison trap to undermine your contentment? Have comparisons led you to desire what is popular rather than what is best? Has focusing on the blessings of others caused you to become ungrateful for your own blessings? Has focusing on God's plan for others caused you to neglect His plan for your life? How can you avoid the curse of comparison in your life?

NOTE

1. William J. Bennett, *The Book of Virtues* (New York: Simon & Schuster, 1993), 213–15.

Chapter Nine *"First the gesture, then the grace."*

THE GIFT
OF GRATITUDE

He who forgets the language of gratitude can never be on speaking terms with happiness. C. Neil Strait

T wo men were walking through an open field when they spotted an enraged bull. Instantly they darted toward the nearest fence. The storming bull followed in hot pursuit, and it was soon apparent that they wouldn't make it. Terrified, one shouted to the other, "Put up a prayer, John. We're in for it!"

John answered, "I can't. I've never made a public prayer in my life."

"But you must!" implored his companion. "The bull is catching up on us."

"All right," panted John, "I'll say the only prayer I know. My father used to repeat it at the table: 'O Lord, for what we are about to receive, make us truly grateful.'"

John's prayer highlights a profound principle: Even the bad things of life improve when we couch them in thanksgiving. A grateful heart is like Mary Poppins's famous spoonful of sugar—it helps the medicine go down in the most delightful way!

Gratitude is not just a gift to God or those to whom we express our appreciation. It is also a gift to us! I am convinced that the Lord instructed us to be thankful for our benefit, not only for His. Gratitude is like a beautifully wrapped package with a big bow on top, ready to be opened by anyone who wants to rise to a new level of living.

It is impossible to be grateful and discontent at the same moment; the two are mutually exclusive. The opposite is also true. It is impossible to be both content and ungrateful at once; one quickly overtakes the other. But it is not a contest of equals. Since our natural tendency is to become complacent or to complain, contentment is usually the loser.

In her autobiographical book *The Hiding Place*, Corrie ten Boom gives a riveting example of the spiritual power of a grateful attitude. Her sister, Betsie, insisted on thanking God for even the apparently negative circumstances in their barracks—the fleas, for example. Betsie insisted that they thank God for the critters. It wasn't until weeks afterward that Betsie discovered the presence of the fleas protected the prisoners. The guards did not want to enter the barracks because of the fleas. So the prisoners could have a Bible study without interference from the guards![1]

Misery is the natural outgrowth of an ungrateful heart. Unfortunately, no matter how good or bad their specific circumstances may become, people who see the worst in every situation will most likely remain miserable people. As C. Neil Strait put it, "Attitudes sour in the life that is closed to thankfulness. Soon selfish attitudes take over, closing life to better things." Of course, the converse is also true. The good things of life take root in soil which has been fertilized with a healthy dose of gratitude.

THE HAVES OR THE HAVE-NOTS

True contentment has more to do with appreciating what we've got than getting what we want. It is not about money or status. It is about attitude and outlook—both of which improve with a spirit of thanksgiving. Therefore, the best gift we can give ourselves is not possession or position, but gratitude.

Beth lives in a small rented house with only a kerosene heater to provide expensive, inefficient, and potentially dangerous heat. The lock on her front door is more for appearance than for security; a child could force the door open. The light in her bathroom does not work, nor do many of the house's outlets. But the house is all Beth can afford with the money she makes at her graveyard-shift service-station job. Beth is working toward better circumstances, but for the moment she has to stay where she is. She says simply, "I've learned not to complain." She has learned to look at what she has rather than what she doesn't have.

But I Don't Feel Grateful

We usually get the whole gratitude experience backwards. We wait until we feel thankful before we give thanks. But gratitude is not a feeling, it is a choice. Like physical exercise, it requires a conscious decision to get moving. Once we develop the habit, however, the benefits motivate us to continue.

The thing we fail to understand is that thankful feelings don't cause us to express gratitude. Rather, expressing gratitude causes us to feel thankful. If we wait until the feelings come, we will never start.

The natural pattern of the human experience is to become complacent. Our brains are wired to sort out things that aren't threatening, harmful, or unique and put them in a "normal experience" category. This allows us to grow accustomed to the more common aspects of living, helping us assimilate the new and exciting into the everyday of life.

Unfortunately, this natural occurrence has a negative edge. It doesn't take long for us to begin taking for granted things once considered exceptional. The television set, for example, was an exciting novelty to my grandparents. But my kids see it as just another piece of furniture. The microwave oven, something I never heard of as a child, now sits in every kitchen and office break room. As a result, I take it for granted.

Think of how many things fall into this category of life—your house, your car, your loved ones, your senses. Imagine how excited you would be to be given the sense of sight if you had been blind since birth. But if you have always been able to see, you may take it for granted. Remember how excited you were to spend time with that special guy or girl before you married the person? Now you complain over his or her minor flaws. Why? Because you take your mate for granted.

For most of us, the feelings of gratitude don't come in proportion to the number of things which we have to be grateful for. Though surrounded by the blessings of life, we can't see them.

143

The good news is that we can counteract this natural tendency toward complacency. How? By consciously choosing gratitude. By counting our blessings, one by one. By saying "thank You" to the giver of all good gifts. Once we begin the process, it is amazing how quickly the thankful feelings come—along with an overwhelming sense of contentment. We suddenly feel wealthy.

Like Magic

Am I suggesting that thankfulness has some kind of magical power to transform our lives and lift our spirits, regardless of circumstance? Yes, I am. Ask anyone who has made an intentional effort to replace complacency with gratitude and you will hear that something dramatic takes place inside. It can seem like magic. But there are some very practical principles at work which help explain why gratitude has such a powerful impact upon our lives.

PRINCIPLE #1: Gratitude shifts our focus from what's wrong to what's right.

William Temple was right. He said, "Man is born crying, lives complaining, and dies disappointed." We spend our lives so consumed with what's wrong, we never seem to enjoy what's right. What a waste!

We all know people who could be labeled "snivelers." You intentionally avoid asking the simple question "How are you?" because they'll take the opportunity to spend thirty minutes moaning and groaning over the trials and tribulations of life.

Perhaps you've heard about the woman who was obsessed with the minor aches and pains of her body. She went to the doctor's office to have her condition diagnosed. The doctor read down a list of potential symptoms.

"Headaches?"

"Yes." she replied.

"Back pain?"

"Yes."

"Sinus trouble?"

"Yes."

This went on for several minutes. She responded affirmatively to every ailment he listed. Finally, the doctor decided to throw out a bizarre symptom just to make a point.

"Do your teeth itch?" he probed, certain she would react to the ridiculous suggestion.

"Well," she said, sliding her tongue across her front teeth, "now that you mention it . . ."

To one degree or another, we all fall into this same trap. We become so accustomed to focusing on the negative things that we begin assuming the worst. Sure, a lot is wrong with this life. There is sickness, heartache, death, poverty, abuse. . . . The list could go on and on. I am not suggesting that we ignore the negative aspects of living. But let's face it. We can become so focused on the bad that we no longer even see the good. That is an extreme we must learn to avoid.

The key is to develop a discipline of gratitude. Think about it. Before we can say "thanks" we must zero in on the things for which we are thankful. And in the process of pondering the positive, we take a much-needed break from contemplating the negative. That's not denial. It's maintaining a healthy perspective—something we could all use.

PRINCIPLE #2: Gratitude shifts our focus off ourselves and onto God.

I'm sure you've heard the lines before:

"Get in touch with your inner self."

"I need to find myself."

"Discover the child within."

"How do you feel about . . . ?"

"I can't love others until I learn to love myself."

"I'm seeking self-actualization."

Each of these phrases contains an element of truth. But they also reveal an unhealthy trend in our society. We are becoming consumed with ourselves. Although there is a place for introspection and self-awareness, we have gone to an extreme with both. We've made "me" the primary focus of life. And in the process of pursuing self-fulfillment, we've taken our eyes off the only One who can give it—God.

The Bible is filled with songs of praise and expressions of thanksgiving directed to God. This is not because He needs it, but because the simple act of expressing appreciation to God for who He is and what He has done helps us keep a proper perspective on our place in the world. We are not the beginning and end of all things. We are the beneficiary, not the source. We are the recipient, not the producer. We are dependent, not independent. We are part of His wonderful plan; He is not part of ours. In short, God is in control—and we aren't. So relax!

Actually, the Scriptures tell us that ingratitude is one symptom of a life which has become consumed with futile and foolish pursuits: "For although they knew God, they neither glorified him as God *nor gave thanks to him,* but their thinking became futile and their foolish hearts were darkened" (Romans 1:21, italics added).

When we neglect the discipline of thanksgiving, our thinking becomes warped. Self takes the throne, and contentment leaves the room. Remember, true contentment is fostered when we trust God, not when we gratify ourselves.

The apostle Paul made the connection between giving thanks to God and having a healthy perspective quite clear. He said,

> Do not be anxious about anything, but in everything, by prayer and petition, *with thanksgiving,* present your requests to God. (Philippians 4:6)

> Let the peace of Christ rule in your hearts, since as members of one body you were called to peace. *And be thankful.* (Colossians 3:15, italics added)

Show me a person who regularly gives thanks, and I'll show you someone who is not preoccupied with himself. I'll also show you a person who has mastered the art of contentment.

PRINCIPLE #3: Gratitude shifts our focus from "what I deserve" to "what I've received."

An attitude of entitlement is the quickest way to sour an otherwise sweet spirit. Yet it is precisely the attitude we are quick to embrace.

"I have my rights!"

"I deserve the best."

"That's not fair!"

"Give me, give me, give me . . ."

We sound like selfish children arguing over the same toy. We want what we want, when we want it. Very unattractive, certainly. But what else did we expect? After all, many of us were spoonfed and pampered since birth. From the first moments of life we got what we wanted by screaming and whining. Unfortunately, though we outgrew the bottles and diapers, we held onto the whining routine.

"Thirtysomething" character Hope Steadman summarized our problem well. "I think our parents got together in 1946 and said, 'Let's have lots of kids and give them everything they want, so that they can grow up and be totally messed up and unable to cope with life.'"

We can't cope with life because we are caught in a perpetual cycle of demanding what we deserve, only to discover that it isn't enough. We are not unhappy because we have it so bad. We are unhappy because we expect so much.

A thankful heart is a satisfied heart. Gratitude shifts our focus from "give me what I deserve" to "look at how much I've received." The former grows out of pride—viewing ourselves as the center of the universe. The latter breeds humility—the realization that we are dependent upon God's goodness. If you have your health, it is not because you deserve health, but because God has given it to you. If you have money, it is not because you deserve money, but because God has given you the ability to make a living. If you have a happy family, it is not because you deserve a happy family, but because God has placed people in your life who love you and whom you love in return.

In short, all good gifts come from God. So instead of demanding what you deserve, try saying thank you for what you've been given.

PRINCIPLE #4: Gratitude shifts us from a paradigm of complacency to a paradigm of praise.

I know, I know. The word "paradigm" has been used by everyone from new age gurus to business revolutionaries, all trying to sell another worn-out concept by packaging it in fancy jargon. But there are proper places for its use—and this is one of them.

A paradigm is nothing more than the way we view the world—
the lens through which we see and assimilate our environment. It
helps us sift through and sort out all of the stuff our brains take in
and place everything in a pre-defined box of understanding. If something doesn't fit into one of our boxes, we either disregard it or create
and label a new box. So a paradigm is like a fence—keeping some
things in and other things out. That can be either good or bad.

Unfortunately, many of us are trapped in a habit of complacency.
We have learned to take for granted the countless wonderful things
around us. We just don't notice them anymore. Our paradigm fence
has kept them outside its borders.

Somehow, we need to break free from the old and begin viewing the world through a new set of lenses. We need to develop and
maintain a paradigm of praise—one which opens our eyes to the
blessings of life, we have either forgotten or taken for granted. One
which takes our focus off the things we lack and places it on the
things we have. One which renews our sense of excitement over the
blessings of life, both big and small. In short, we need to become
grateful.

When we thank God for the blessings of life, whether or not we
feel like it, something happens to our perspective. It lifts us above the
pettiness of "poor me" and helps us view life from a higher vantage
point. I believe one of the reasons King David was called "a man
after God's own heart" (see 1 Samuel 13:14) is that he had discovered and mastered the art of thanksgiving. He intentionally fostered a
spirit of gratitude. He routinely reminded himself and others of God's
goodness. He intentionally, verbally, creatively, and enthusiastically
voiced his praise to God. As a result, he learned to see the best in
every circumstance—even the bad. David's words reveal the paradigm through which he saw life.

> Enter his gates with thanksgiving, and his courts with praise; give
> thanks to him and praise his name. For the Lord is good and his love
> endures forever; his faithfulness continues through all generations.
> (Psalm 100:4–5)

> Give thanks to the Lord, for he is good; his love endures forever.
> (Psalm 106:1)

THE GIFT OF GRATITUDE

Let them give thanks to the Lord for his unfailing love and his wonderful deeds for men. Let them sacrifice thank offerings and tell of his works with songs of joy. (Psalm 107:21–22)

Why are you downcast, O my soul? Why so disturbed within me? Put your hope in God, for I will yet praise him, my Savior and my God. (Psalm 43:5)

For God is the King of all the earth; sing to him a psalm of praise. (Psalm 47:7)

Let everything that has breath praise the Lord. Praise the Lord. (Psalm 150:6)

Some of these powerful praise sessions took place when everything was going wrong, when David's whole world seemed to be falling apart. Yet, David consciously chose to view life through a paradigm of praise. As a result, he was able to maintain a healthy perspective both in times of blessing and in times of pain.

Let's face it. We all need the kind of refreshment which comes from an occasional vacation on the island of appreciation. Go ahead. Give it a try. I guarantee the trip will lift your spirits and alter your attitude. I'm sure you could use a bit of both.

Getting Personal

H ave you ever tried to be grateful and discontent at the same moment? What are some practical ways you can develop the discipline of thanksgiving in your life? How can you shift your focus off yourself and onto God? Go ahead, give yourself the best gift of all—gratitude.

NOTE

1. Corrie ten Boom with John and Elizabeth Sherrill, *The Hiding Place* (Grand Rapids: Chosen, 1971), 181, 190.

Chapter Ten

MAKING
OURSELVES RICH

There are people who have money and people who are rich. Coco Gabrielle Chanel

I f the best way to make a man poor is to increase his wants, then the best way to make him rich is to show him the path to contentment. That is precisely what I have attempted to do. My goal has been to help you examine and apply life principles which can foster a spirit of contentment in the midst of a world that has confused the definition of happiness . . . to make yourself rich by discovering the natural wealth of contentment.

We live in the lovely little town of Colorado Springs, Colorado. Though too small to host a major-league baseball team, we do have our very own minor-league club, the Colorado Springs Sky Sox. Sky Sox stadium is located on the outskirts of town, where thousands of loyal fans watch their favorite not-quite-big-league players compete for the win . . . and a shot at the majors. The atmosphere at a minor-league baseball game is less intense and more relaxed than it is in the big leagues. Fans have a lot of fun, especially when the park does something special, or crazy, to boost attendance.

A good friend of mine recently attended just such a day at the park with her twelve-year-old daughter, Danielle. It was Mother's Day 1994, and the ballpark was hosting an on-field treasure hunt at the end of the game. A small treasure chest had been buried somewhere under the infield, and mothers and daughters were invited to team up and dig for it. Now, under normal circumstances, these ladies would have snubbed their noses at such an undignified suggestion. But they knew that the treasure chest contained a very special prize . . . a diamond ring! So, hundreds of otherwise elegant women were in attendance, eagerly waiting for the game to end so that they could begin scratching and clawing through mounds of dirt in search of a girl's best friend.

Danielle and her mother were among the participants. Gardening shovels in hand, they walked out onto the field and began digging through the dirt along with the others. It was a frantic scene. Dirt was flying everywhere as the search began. Several of the more aggressive women gave new meaning to the phrase "survival of the fittest." "Get out of my way, kid!" yelled one woman. "Hey, that's my spot!" shouted another. Children were trampled over if they happened to get in the way. Everyone wanted that ring, and they were willing to lose all dignity and decency in order to get it.

After only a few minutes, Danielle's tiny shovel hit something near third base where she had been digging. She quickly pushed away the surrounding dirt and pulled free a small box in the shape of a treasure chest. Noticing her discovery, the host ran toward Danielle and proclaimed her the winner of the treasure hunt. Jealous faces all around made it clear that the others were anything but excited for this sweet little girl who had robbed them of their prize.

The host gathered everyone together to watch Danielle open the treasure chest. All eyes were glued to her as she popped open the lid and revealed the coveted ring. It was exquisite! Catching a sunbeam, the ring glittered and sparkled—intensifying the disappointment of those who lost. Danielle had a big grin on her face, clutching tightly to the treasure chest she had won.

As the crowd dispersed, Danielle and her mother began to walk away. But the host stopped them. "Excuse me, honey," he called. "The ring is yours. But I need to keep the treasure chest to use again later." He tried to pull it from her hands, but he sensed some resistance. Danielle's mother watched her daughter's grin dissolve.

"Can I have the box, sweetie?" the host persisted.

"OK," came Danielle's response.

As she and her mother drove home from the game, Danielle sat in silence. Her mother looked over at her with a smile. "You really wanted to keep the treasure chest, didn't you, honey?"

"I sure did. I would have given back the ring if he would have just let me keep the treasure chest," Danielle admitted. "I really liked that treasure chest."

"Are you disappointed?" Mom inquired.

"Well, I guess not. After all, I did win a diamond ring!"

Hundreds of women practically killed to get that diamond ring. Yet Danielle was more impressed with the ten-dollar plastic box. The others were bitter over a kid getting what they wanted. Yet she was willing to give back the ring in order to keep the treasure chest. I for one think that Danielle had the right idea.

Danielle's treasure chest is a wonderful picture of what it is to discover natural wealth. While everyone else loses all perspective in pursuit of artificial riches (the diamond ring), we can experience the simple joys of content living (the plastic box). In childish simplicity, Danielle has taught us well the key to contentment. You see, the secret is not in acquiring the treasure. It is rather in learning to enjoy the box. But how? To answer that question, we'll have to return to the car and listen to the rest of the conversation.

"Mom, while we were standing on the field getting ready to search for the ring, I prayed a prayer."

"And what did you pray, honey?" asked Danielle's mom.

"I asked the Lord to let me find the diamond ring. But that even if I didn't find it, that He would let us all have a good time looking anyway."

Let's glean from Danielle's simple wisdom. God may or may not give us the treasure we seek. But even if He doesn't, He can help us have a good time anyway! And that, my friends, is contentment in a nutshell. We can't always control our circumstances, but God can. Being content where He has placed us, being grateful for the good He has given us, and working to improve what He allows us to change—these are the keys to lessening the burden of life's expectations and the essence of traveling light.